Dr Aric Sigman specialises in child health education. He is a
Fellow of The Society of Biology and Associate Fellow of The
British Psychological Society. His health and psychology book

Gettir

Inforn

aspect

Thins

Britaii

Educa

The S

public

variou

Turkn

Iran,

Sumat

For m

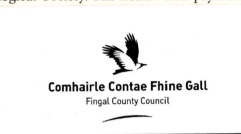

Also by Dr Aric Sigman

Remotely Controlled
The Spoilt Generation
Alcohol Nation

The
Body
Wars

Why body dissatisfaction is
at epidemic proportions and
how we can fight back

Dr Aric Sigman

piatkus

PIATKUS

First published in Great Britain in 2014 by Piatkus

A CIP catalogue record for this book
is available from the British Library.

ISBN 978-0-349-40128-7

Note for the reader
The recommendations in this book are intended solely
as education and information. This book is not intended as a substitute for
professional medical care in cases of serious Body Dysmorphic Disorder or eating
disorders. If you think you or one of your family members has a problem with
Body Dysmorphic Disorder or any other eating disorder, seek medical help
from your doctor or equivalent health professional.

P.64 © Nadine Gordimer, The Pickup, Bloomsbury Publishing Plc.
P.73 'Everybody Needs a Bosom for a Pillow' © Tjinder Singh.

Typeset in Sabon by M Rules
Printed and bound in Great Britain by
Clays Ltd, St Ives plc

Papers used by Piatkus are from well-managed forests
and other responsible sources.

Contents

Acknowledgements   vii
Preface   ix

PART ONE

1   Size Matters   3
2   Know Your Wiggle Room   22
3   A Source of Thinspiration   44
4   What Men Want   64
5   Baby Dissatisfaction   87
6   Manorexia   102

PART TWO
The Shape of Things to Come

7   Paradigm Shift   123
8   Running Away from Body Dissatisfaction   135
9   Well Connected?   145
10 Altered Images   160
11 In Our Own Image   166
12 Downsizing   183
13 War and Peace   198

Appendix   208
References   214
Resources   245
Further Reading   248
Index   250

Acknowledgements

The women in my life, comprising several generations – from my daughters to my mother – have all been immensely helpful in forming and refining my ideas on how women feel about their bodies. To her credit, my editor Anne Lawrance saw that there was a different way to look at body dissatisfaction and that men's views on the matter are relevant. Moreover, she didn't try to coax me into adopting a predictable, comfy 'learn-to-celebrate-your-body' approach to this subject. My agent Sara Menguc not only aided and abetted the commissioning of the book but provided marvellous insights into how even the most accomplished, intelligent women can still be competitive dieters. For the third book now, my copy-editor Anne Newman has reined in my excesses, checked my logic and saved me from clumsily insulting as many people as I might otherwise have done; she confidently second-guessed my intentions, making the editing process for me far easier than it should have been. My wife Katy has had the pleasure of enduring endless discussions on, among other things, the joyful cardiometabolic benefits of gluteofemoral fat, the fascinating functional differences between brown and white fat, followed by the extraordinary significance of the foetal programming and epigenetics of body composition; she then had free, unlimited twenty-four-hour access to my withering views on famous people and their diets.

Preface

Over the many years I've been involved in health education, there's one issue straddling both mental and physical health that, given its abstract nature, has proved elusive and intractable: body image. Alcohol is a substance – amounts can be measured, and so can the consequences. Yet while we can grasp anorexia because we can see people becoming thinner and can measure their weight loss, getting our teeth into what a 'poor body image' actually is, what 'body dissatisfaction' means and what difference it makes to people's lives hasn't been straightforward. The idea that our own perceptions of how we look can translate into profound mental and physical changes involves too many indistinct links in a long and winding chain for it to be fully understood and taken as seriously as it should be. And given other more immediate, high-profile health issues, the way people feel about their body size and shape seems a mild concern in comparison.

  You may wonder why a man should be so bothered about the way girls and women feel about their bodies. My concerns are part professional – I spend a great deal of my time trying to reduce body dissatisfaction and prevent unnecessary dieting and the development of eating disorders in girls and women. But I'm also a father. The prospect of my daughters being culturally bullied and browbeaten into assuming that they're overweight, unattractive and unworthy makes me angry. Visions of a Clint Eastwood style of summary justice come to mind, whereby today's body-image bandits – a veritable rogues' gallery of the media's casting directors, producers, directors, commissioning and picture editors responsible for a crime spree of body dissatisfaction, along with 'hate crimes' against size-16s – are lined up. But instead of being tarred and feathered, they'd be forced to remove all clothing and make-up and marched naked along the catwalks of New York, London, Paris, Milan and Tokyo, in full glare of the cameras, to reveal their own humanity in all its glory – be it cellulite, moobs or even more than just the one chin. Unfortunately, however, it seems this doesn't comply with the UN Bill of Human Rights – so I've resorted to writing this book instead.

Women's sensitivity about their bodies was something I, as one of five boys, didn't understand until well into adulthood. My late cousin was a bigshot in the fashion industry – Ralph Lauren, Tommy Hilfiger, Donna Karan and even Sean 'P. Diddy' Combs were at his memorial service – and while on the fashion-show circuit he'd come to London and would take me out to dinner with his entourage of svelte designers and catwalk models. A devoted gourmand, he frequented *very* good restaurants, and I, being young and hungry, would order and eat as much as possible with no shame. But I recall how the slenderati at the table – the models in particular – would order little and leave a lot on their plates. With few manners and little self-consciousness, I'd routinely lighten their burden by reaching across the table and finishing off their filet mignon, scallops and lobster, along with their look-but-don't-touch decadent puddings. It was a marvellous arrangement: they seemed grateful to have been relieved of temptation, while I'd eat two or three dinners for the price of none. I was clearly more interested in the food than I was in the models (who, in retrospect, seemed utterly sexless). In fact, come to think of it, all of those fashionistas seemed acutely aware of what and how they ate and the effect it could have on their appearance; they were also very aware of how others around them looked, and I remember one of them commenting about a cele/deb entering the room, 'But she's a [size] ten,' in less than flattering tones.

I've since discovered that many women don't like others to see 'the numbers' – their weight or their dress size. I've noticed that at the checkout women often prefer those queuing not to see the size of the dress they are buying, for example. However, true enlightenment came when I was first asked, 'Does this dress make me look fat?' and learned, very quickly, that George Washington's counsel (that honesty is always the best policy) was not altogether helpful – you don't reply truthfully, 'No, darling. It's your *fat* that makes you look fat.'

In trying to understand the world of female body image, what has been most astonishing is how even the most intelligent, capable, rational and 'empowered' women I've known, loved, worked with and for, can be laid low by body dissatisfaction. This includes women with body shapes a man would die for. Most men assume that an otherwise confident woman wouldn't be bothered that deeply by something as superficial as a bit of fat or a patch of cellulite. Many of us just don't get it.

And so when it comes to the world of women's body image, eating disorders and dieting, there has been a distinct lack of male input. It has understandably been dominated almost entirely by women. However, for better or worse, we are inextricably entwined: half of all fathers have daughters, 90 per cent of men will have a wife/partner; we also have mothers, sisters and female friends. Therefore, men have a big stake in female body dissatisfaction and not only are we entitled to comment, we are now required to storm in and say something to help change the ways the girls and women in our lives feel about their bodies. This should not be misconstrued or wilfully misinterpreted as a patronising, paternalistic overture to rescue poor, inept, defenceless women. (And, as you will see, men too have more than their fair share of body dissatisfaction and need help from women to overcome it.)

One of the reasons for men's lack of involvement in this issue is that instead of being considered a source of help to women's body image, heterosexual men have traditionally been cited as the cause of the problem. Women's body woes and wars were, and according to some still are, the fault of 'the male gaze', a product of heterosexual male demands for the diet-induced, slender female bodies we are told men desire and expect. But as you will see in Chapter 4, 'What Men Want', men actually have a very different and much kinder take on female body fat, sex appeal, eating and weight loss than they're given credit for. Hetero men may indeed be guilty of many things, including the sexual objectification of women and of fuelling the breast-enlargement craze. But the growing disdain for the pear shape – and female body fat around hips, thighs and bottoms in general – is quite a different matter. And trying to explain it away with tried-and-tested explanations of sexism is no longer sufficient, nor is it constructive.

And so this book, among other things, calls on the untapped army of men – husbands, partners, fathers and brothers – to enlist, and support women in facing down this modern-day demon, to prevent and reduce what is, in effect, a worldwide epidemic of body dissatisfaction, so as to enable women and girls to live longer and more fulfilling lives.

The driving forces behind body dissatisfaction are widespread, ranging from the media, our culture and our own deeply embedded emotions, values and judgments about our bodies to our biological predispositions. In tackling this we're also going to have to confront today's established slender norms promoted by multi-billion-dollar industries that continue to perpetuate and profit from the level of body dissatisfaction they've managed to bring about. There are obviously no instant self-help cures for body dissatisfaction because many of the necessary changes are cultural, financial and political and beyond our immediate control. And so to suggest that reading a book will cause you to 'love your body' is pure fantasy of the kind offered up in the very magazines that have helped cause body dissatisfaction to begin with. However, there is a great deal we can do as individuals to significantly lessen the effects of body dissatisfaction, enabling us to lead less troubled, healthier and more fulfilling lives: to feel more comfortable with our size and shape. As parents there's a great deal we can do to prevent our children from experiencing body dissatisfaction the way our generation has.

As a first port of call this book will survey the state we're in: the sheer extent of body dissatisfaction today, its potential causes and its many consequences that few are aware of. Pregnancy and the look of motherhood has increasingly become a source of heightened body dissatisfaction, it's highly revealing to try and understand how and why. I feel it's imperative to understand our own bodies before we consider being dissatisfied with them. And so I've provided an overview of the factors that influence our body shape and weight along with a slightly more scientific understanding of our sadly misunderstood and much hated, body fat. It's also important that we try to fully understand the enemy without and within to enable us to fight back and change things for the better. For example to familiarise ourselves with some of the mechanisms which enable the media to literally alter the way our brains function along with the way we feel about ourselves, so significantly. It's useful to see female body dissatisfaction from a very different perspective by looking at how men express their body dissatisfaction.

Ultimately we must try to take control of the areas of our lives that we can influence for the better in ways that will indirectly and directly improve the way we feel about our own bodies. Beyond a mere understanding of body dissatisfaction I've gone on to present a veritable pot pourri of tangible things we as individuals and as parents can do to improve matters. And finally there are institutional changes recommended for schools, media and government. But, in the here and now, fighting back against the recent tide of body dissatisfaction requires foot soldiers.

Let the battle begin ...

PART ONE

One

Size Matters

Forty years after the debut of body politics, fat is more of a feminist issue than ever. Whether fat or slender, girls and women of all ages have never been so unhappy with their bodies. And underweight women are often no more satisfied with their body weight than those who are overweight. In our society, perversely, it is now abnormal for a woman to be content with her body shape.

In the name of aspiring to be 'fit and toned', body dissatisfaction has become so prevalent among girls and women that it is now being described as 'a normative discontent'. It is insidious and pervasive. And it's appearing at younger and younger ages. Nearly half of the three- to six-year-old girls in a study in the *British Journal of Developmental Psychology* said they worry about being fat.[1]

What's more, it seems that worry doesn't diminish with age: a preoccupation with physique and body dissatisfaction is now found even among a high proportion of pensioners.[2] A large study in the *International Journal of Eating Disorders* found that 8 per cent of women over fifty, including those over seventy-five, have made themselves vomit in the last five years.[3] Furthermore, there is also growing alarm over school-aged *boys* taking anabolic steroids to build muscle and acquire a six-pack.[4]

Globally, body dissatisfaction has made a startling debut and seems assured a long run on the world stage. The first International Body Project recently published their report on female body dissatisfaction 'in 26 Countries Across 10 World Regions' and concluded, 'body dissatisfaction and desire for thinness is commonplace', emphasising 'the need for international attention to this problem'.[5] And global body dissatisfaction is contagious: international data from the World Health Organization's survey 'Health Behaviour in School-aged Children' reveal a high level of body dissatisfaction, triggering 'significant health concerns among health professionals worldwide'.[6]

Looking ahead, fewer and fewer young women will ever have known a time when it wasn't completely normal for the average woman to be unhappy with her body. And as they enter positions of influence in the media, body dissatisfaction is becoming the normal baseline from which media and society operate. As the commissioning editor of the *Observer* magazine writes: 'To be feminine, today, means to hate your body.'[7]

Size matters more than ever, it seems, and whether you're genuinely obese or one of the slim 'worried well' who *feels* larger than life, keeping up appearances is getting us down.

But why has it become normal to dislike your own body from age three? Why are eating disorders and weight and shape concerns affecting so many women? And what can we do to deal with the negative effects this is having on people's lives?

Effects

Body dissatisfaction is more than an uncomfortable feeling about being seen in a swimsuit or harbouring the nagging question, 'Does this dress make me look fat?' The effects can be wide-ranging, long-lasting and fatal. Those involved in the treatment of diabetes are concerned that body dissatisfaction leads to poor control of patients' blood-sugar levels.[8] And studies now report that body dissatisfaction 'has a strong impact on all suicidal behaviors for girls', even when they are not overweight: because it's not about actual weight, but about *perception*.[9]

Sex, cigs and booze

Women may drink to feel comfortable with the way they think their bodies look, and many girls smoke for a more slim-line appearance.[10] A study of 81,000 adolescents by the Division of Epidemiology, University of Minnesota found that 'smoking for weight control is prevalent'.[11] Scientists can predict the likelihood of a girl smoking in the future by how important it is for her to be thin today.[12] And by the time they're young women a relationship can be formed whereby smoking and drinking increase right along with body dissatisfaction.[13]

Sexual health and taking sexual risks are also linked to body dissatisfaction, as reflected in the study 'Early Adolescent Body Image Predicts Subsequent Condom Use Behavior Among Girls'.[14] And those who feel least attractive tend to be most prone to engaging in relatively risky sexual behaviour. One explanation is that when a person feels like the less attractive partner in a couple, he or she has less leverage or power within that relationship and is, therefore, vulnerable to allowing the 'more attractive' partner to instigate risky sexual behaviour. Another suspicion is that less attractive people have fewer sexual encounters and, therefore, less practice at negotiating safer sexual behaviour with a partner. And some suggest that if you have lower body satisfaction, the degree of excitement and arousal experienced when you're faced with pending sexual activity with a partner you think is far more attractive than you can result in more impulsive decision making.[15]

Inactivity

It has been suggested that regular exercise can reduce the risk of breast cancer by as much as a third.[16] Yet many young women say they are simply too embarrassed about their bodies to ever be seen exercising. Britain's mental health charity Mind surveyed women and found that 90 per cent of those over thirty 'battle body-confidence and low self-esteem when considering outdoor exercise. This is leading many to take extreme measures, such as exercising when it's dark to minimise embarrassment, or to avoid outdoor activities altogether.'[17]

Academic achievement

At the cerebral end of concerns, body dissatisfaction in university students has a strong link with 'academic interference' and lower grades.[18] It's thought that body dissatisfaction may lead students to be preoccupied with and to 'monitor' their bodies' appearance which, in turn, uses up their attention and intellectual resources, making these unavailable for answering the questions on an exam paper. It sounds like a slapstick comedy approach to research, but two studies looked at the performance of women on a maths exam, based on what they were wearing: one group was asked to strip down to just swimsuits, while the others wore sweaters. The swimwear-clad women performed significantly worse in the exam than their covered-up counterparts because, it's thought, they were partially distracted by monitoring their body instead of the equations in front of them.[19]

Non-academic achievement

Those women aspiring to a more physical career in baseball, rounders or cricket may be interested in the study 'Throwing Like A Girl: Self-Objectification Predicts Adolescent Girls' Motor Performance'. Being concerned about body appearance was related to girls' ability to throw a softball, even after other factors were controlled for. Again, the diversion of the girls' attention towards how their bodies looked as opposed to the task of throwing the ball seemed to result in less forceful throws and poorer aim.[20]

Professional achievement

When women do complete their education there is concern that body dissatisfaction holds them back professionally. Women who are more likely to internalise the views of others, including the media, may actually feel less capable than those who put less emphasis on appearance.[21] In an image-driven culture where body shape and dress sense count big, women may feel disempowered and not put themselves forward. An 'Analysis of the Political Effects of Self-Objectification' carried out at Occidental College in California found that the more women self-objectify (monitor their bodies' appearance), 'the less confidence they have that their actions have the potential to influence politics … they may be less likely to vote or run for office'.[22]

The media eye, in its various forms, objectifies all of us. And so many of us begin to objectify ourselves. If women are insecure about and busy monitoring their bodies' appearance this may be a self-perpetuating behaviour preventing them from making enough of a fuss about our society's values which contribute to them feeling bad about their bodies to begin with.[23]

Relationships

Our relationships – both platonic and otherwise – may be affected by the way we feel about our bodies. Body dissatisfaction can unknowingly erode friendships through what is referred to as 'dieting peer competitiveness' – and there's even a scale to measure it: the DPC Scale.[24] Greater body dissatisfaction has been 'linked to less secure general attachment, especially more preoccupied general adult attachment and more anxious romantic attachment'. It's also associated with 'interpersonal anxiety' and with 'romantic intimacy anxiety' for women.[25]

Sexual satisfaction

Sexologists and body-image scientists have mated, giving birth to some interesting findings. Body-image concerns are now linked to 'lower sexual arousability and ability to reach orgasm and less pleasure from physical intimacy', which is thought to be due to the insidious influence of our slim image-driven culture joining us under the duvet.[26] And distraction rears its ugly head here again too. A woman's degree of body dissatisfaction is found to be strongly related to how distracted she becomes during sex, both in terms of her concerns over the way she looks or how she is 'performing' in bed.[27] The distracting effects of a woman's body image on achievement during a maths exam (see p. 6) has a lot in common with those on a very different type of achieving: orgasms.[28] On the other hand, women who are more satisfied with their bodies report having more frequent orgasms, as well as 'trying new sexual behaviors'.[29] Yes, yes, yes ... There are body-image scientists who keep count of these things.

On the whole, a large proportion of women, both heterosexual and lesbian, say that the way they feel about their bodies has a negative effect on the enjoyment of their sex lives and how desirable they feel they are as a sexual partner.[30]

Those who assume that women who are satisfied with their bodies and therefore enjoying sex more are obviously slimmer or exercise more and are, therefore, 'fit and toned' may be interested in the findings of one study that looked at precisely this. While Body Mass Index (see p. 34) and level of physical exercise had no bearing on 'sexual functioning', women with low body dissatisfaction had 'high sexual assertiveness and sexual esteem, low sexual anxiety, and fewer sexual problems'.[31] And another study brought women into the lab who completed measures of body-image concerns and were then exposed to 'erotica', while their genital responses were monitored by the researchers. 'Body esteem was positively related to sexual desire, including desire to erotica in a laboratory setting and as well as desire in real-life sexual situations, outside of the contrived laboratory setting ... independent of actual body size.'[32]

Causes

What factors can possibly lead us to be less than happy about our bodies? Below are a variety of interesting suspects.

Fat friends, pear-shaped peers

Although there is an increasing understanding of the role of the media underlying the dramatic growth in body dissatisfaction, new research is shedding light on the role of our own best friends in the contagious spread of our body concerns.

Some researchers see your friends' body shape acting as a 'catalyst' in triggering body competition with your peers.[33] This body competition and the body dissatisfaction that results from it can arise no matter how close to or fond you are of your friends – or even your husband. Two new studies have looked specifically at your romantic partner's influence on your body image, and it seems Jack Sprat comes out of the comparison feeling pretty good about himself. In love or not, straight or gay, heavier women who had relatively thin partners were most likely to think that they themselves were overweight.[34]

Interestingly, lesbian women may suffer less body dissatisfaction, be more accepting of other women's body size and shapes and actually prefer larger women.[35]

If your friends are fat, it may not be good for their health, but may well be good for yours. In fact, in a new study of women across all EU countries entitled 'Anorexia, Body Image and Peer Effects', researchers found that the fatter your friends are, the less likely you are to be anorexic.[36]

Taking this peer influence even further, it now seems that it isn't merely how fat or slender your friend actually *is*, but how fat or slender you believe she *thinks* she is that can also influence your feelings about your own body. Examining how much of a young woman's body concerns are shaped by her *perceptions* of her friends' concerns with their own bodies versus their *actual* body concerns, researchers found that how women *think* their friends feel about their bodies influences their own body concerns. They also found that the more women felt under pressure to be thin, the more likely they were to have body-image concerns, irrespective of their actual weight and shape. Body dissatisfaction is often literally a process of mind over matter.[37]

Fat talk

The no-beating-about-the-bush study entitled 'If You're Fat, Then I'm Humongous! ... Impact of Fat Talk Among College Women' recently calculated that more than 90 per cent of college-aged women engage in 'fat talk' and 'there was no association between a woman's actual body size and how often she complained about her body size with peers', wrote the scientists. They are concerned that women might think 'fat talk' is a helpful coping mechanism, when it's actually exacerbating body-image disturbance: 'These results serve as a reminder that for most women, fat talk is not about being fat, but rather about feeling fat ... reinforcing women's body-related distress.'[38] A systematic review of the potential effect of talking big in front of your friends reported that 'studies give an initial indication that fat talking is a causal risk factor for body dissatisfaction'.[39] So it seems a problem shared is a problem doubled.

Large print

The books you read may also be influencing body dissatisfaction. While the potential effects of visual media will be discussed in detail in Chapter 3, 'A Source of Thinspiration', researchers are only now examining how the written word may have an effect on your body image. In their study 'Does this book make me look fat?' they found that women's body image can be negatively affected by chick lit. Researchers chose two chick-lit novels – Emily Giffin's *Something Borrowed* and Laura Jensen Walker's *Dreaming in Black and White*, each of which features a heroine with 'healthy body weight', but 'low body esteem'. To observe how a character's weight and body image may affect the reader in different ways they adapted a passage from both novels to come up with nine versions for each, from an underweight heroine with high body esteem to an overweight one with low body esteem – so for example, a character who says, 'I'm five foot four, 140 pounds and a size six', or one who says, 'I'm five foot four, 105 pounds and a size zero'. The study found that when the narrative was about a slim heroine, participants felt significantly less sexually attractive, and that when it featured a protagonist with low body esteem, readers were considerably more concerned about their weight than those in the control condition.[40]

If looks could kill

The great falling out of love with our bodies has been accompanied by the emergence of a fetishistic hunger for all things foodie. Although it's marvellous that we take a greater interest in food, in terms of taste and/or our health, our interest often verges on the unnatural. We're encouraged by food media, celebrity chefs and dieting articles to think about food in preoccupied ways, instead of simply considering it. This has given rise to what some call eating cognitively, whereby food takes on a heightened significance, causing an overemphasis on a part of life that should be less contrived. And while food can be an outlet for creativity, celebration and joy, it can also be misappropriated for expressing other less constructive aspects of the human condition.

I've always felt that generally, men eat food, while women have a relationship with it. And the way you feel about your body can distort that relationship, ultimately providing an entry pass to far greater problems. It is now known to increase your risk of going on to develop an eating disorder such as the newly recognised binge-eating disorder,[41] bulimia and EDNOS (eating disorder not otherwise specified) – a common diagnosis for people with a mixture of atypical anorexia and atypical bulimia.

For some girls and women, the preoccupation with being

slender leads to anorexia nervosa – the UK's deadliest psycholog-ical condition killing more people in Britain than all 'substance misuse' put together.[42] Here's some food for thought:

- The American Psychological Association reported that 'one out of every five people with anorexia eventually dies of causes related to the disorder', and it is linked with one the highest suicide rates of any psychiatric condition.[43]
- The mortality rate associated with anorexia nervosa is twelve times higher than that of *all* causes of death in females aged fifteen to twenty-four years old.[44]
- People first diagnosed with anorexia in their twenties have eighteen times the death risk of healthy people their age.[45]
- Given Britain's current level of anorexia,[46] between 7000 and 14,000 girls and women will ultimately die of anorexia-related causes. This is far greater than the number of women in the UK killed each year through domestic violence or with heterosexually contracted HIV/AIDS.[47]
- In the United States, a conservative estimate indicates that 28,550 girls and women with anorexia will ultimately die as a result of their condition – that's thirteen times more than the total number of American servicemen *and* women killed in the entire Afghan war.[48] While the media has raised a great deal of awareness over the latter, consciousness-raising of death by anorexia has gone missing in action.
- The recent 'Westernisation' of Eastern European countries has led to widespread changes in female ideals and roles that have also increased the risk for eating disorders. For example, in the Czech Republic, a country undergoing a 'socio-cultural transition', the hospital admission rate for eating disorders in females aged ten to thirty-nine has quadrupled, suggesting 'risk of severe eating disorders including anorexia nervosa is culture-dependent'.[49]

- Eating disorders are also on the increase in the non-Western countries previously thought to have greater cultural immunity. A study has found that 'the prevalence of eating disorders among female university students in China is now similar to that of their Western counterparts',[50] while a significant rise is now also reported in Japan.[51]

Each case of an eating disorder involves a complicated background of genetic risk, environmental and social triggers. And for many people with anorexia the underlying psychological problems are still poorly understood. There may be personality traits, such as perfectionism, that in partnership with body dissatisfaction are more likely to set you up for an eating disorder.[52] And the Autism Research Centre at Cambridge University recently found that 'females with anorexia have elevated autistic traits'.[53]

In long-term cases anorexia may not be the result of wanting to be thin or attractive, but rather an attempt to stay in control, a fear of losing control and other feelings. Controlling weight and food intake becomes the unwitting voice through which some women express their psychological pain. So if a culture puts pressure on women to be slim anyway, then their psychological pain may be handed an instruction booklet to funnel itself through food and weight. And after a certain period of time – or degree of weight loss – the eating disorder can take on a life of its own.

If this discussion on eating disorders sounds a bit too relevant to you, there's further information available in the Resources section.

Fit-and-toned Cloak

Psychological pain and/or the desire to be thin can also be channelled through burning the calories at the other end of the candle by over-exercising: engaging in strenuous physical activity to a point that is unsafe and unhealthy. Eating disorders and over-exercising go hand in hand – both can be a result of an unhealthy obsession with your body. Like bulimia and anorexia, in which people deny themselves adequate nutrition by restrictive eating behaviours, over-exercising is a controlled behaviour that denies the body the energy and nutrition needed to maintain a healthy weight.[54]

The most dangerous aspect of over-exercising is how easily it can go unrecognised because it can so readily be disguised as an emphasis on fitness or a desire to be healthy. And in a culture that reveres thin female athletes, lean and mean actresses and singers, and reads 'health and fitness' magazines, a thin woman in Lycra pounding the pavement wearing iPod headphones and a hydration fluid bottle on her hip isn't likely to make us stop and search for clues as to the underlying motivation.

Under the fit-and-toned/healthy-eating guise, many slender, beautiful celebrities perpetuate that unattainable ideal that somehow always seems to be just within your grasp, yet few tell the truth about how they actually achieve it. Some are, however, now doing the right thing; in her article 'What I Wish I'd Said To My Fans' American model and actress Carré Otis reveals the lies she told about her diet and exercise routine:

> 'Jazzercise three times a week and light weights,' I'd say. The heavily guarded truth was that I exercised a minimum of two hours a day, seven days a week . . . my big diet staple was four to six cups of black coffee per day, avoiding even a splash of skim milk since I was terrified of extra calories. And to stave off hunger, I went through a few packs of cigarettes daily.

She recounts the way her exhaustion (a result of lack of sleep, too much exercise, virtual starvation and self-loathing) was hidden beneath a beautiful exterior, made possible by the powers of airbrushing and beauty treatments

> In every shot my fake smile revealed sparkling teeth. Without my on-set manicures and pedicures, you'd have seen that, just like my teeth, my nails were breaking and yellow.[55]

We can only imagine how many other slender dignitaries are currently lying through their airbrushed teeth about their health routines.

The Slenderati

Editors of the successful international women's magazines continue to extol the virtue of their own role in 'empowering' women through their inspiring articles and promotion of 'strong female role models'. They've beaten their chests for decades proclaiming that their mags have helped to liberate women. But the photographs of very slim Photoshopped women they promote in their magazines tell a very different and unchanging story. As you will see, a large body of research is clearly showing that far from empowering women, the pictorial landscape of each edition has merely handed them a new line in shackles.

And it isn't just glossy fashion mags and popular tabloid newspapers. Even serious liberal-left publications with a focus on politics and the arts routinely promoting women's 'equality' and rights regularly feature right-on, edgy designer collections with photos of skinny models and plenty of slender, young images to accompany articles on everything from cucumber salads to bicycles. The slender bent is endemic and apolitical.

Following the path of the food and alcohol industries, the fashion and beauty industry has attempted to airbrush its own image through various 'social responsibility' initiatives. Every couple of years we hear, yet again, how this company or that has decided to include one or two photos of *real* women as part of their celebration of 'real beauty'.

What all publications want to avoid discussing, however, is their addictive need to sell those all-important expensive advertisements, featuring more of the slender. Editors may claim that the pictures in ads are an entirely different matter, but they are certainly not. As so often, it's a case of follow the money. And the trail leads to a dependency on slim images to keep the lifeline of cash flowing from their paymasters: the advertisers.

In an attempt to offset any harm done to women's body image, the fashion, media and beauty industries are now disseminating 'media literacy' materials – videos, booklets and lesson plans – to schools to help girls understand that what they see, say on the pages of a magazine, is artificial. So what they're saying in other words is: when regularly presented with a mosaic of willowy bodies, it's *your* perception that's the underlying problem not the industry that produces them. The subtext being, 'It's not us, it's *you* that needs to change.'

Scientists are increasingly using the 'C'-word – causation – in describing the role of media in the development of eating disorders. In response to the findings of the study of women across all EU countries mentioned above, the recommended solutions are aggressive, urging governments to 'take action to influence role models and compensate for social pressure on women [that is] driving the trade-off between ideal weight and health.'[56]

While both body dissatisfaction and eating disorders may be linked to pre-existing 'lower self-esteem' or the degree to which a woman 'internalises the thin ideal body shape', the culture to which you are exposed can itself lower your self-esteem and cause you to internalise what is on the menu – a platter of underweight images – whether you ordered it or not.

Career Aspirations

Profound changes in our environment, especially if they are rapid, are often accompanied by side effects. Evolutionary adaptation is rarely a comfortable process.

Dr April R. Smith and her colleagues have proposed an intriguing evolutionary explanation of how rising competition between women for professional status – 'intrasexual resource competition' – has inadvertently overstimulated one underlying competitive mechanism between women: changing their body shape and losing weight. In her study 'The pursuit of success: can status aspirations negatively affect body satisfaction?' Smith found that after being exposed to thin, successful women, females with high 'status aspiration' reported significantly worse body satisfaction and greater feelings of ineffectiveness than those with low status aspiration. Historically, she believes, in order to eat and get a roof over their heads and protection, women had to compete for these resources by bagging a good man. But times have certainly changed and women no longer depend on men for survival, often competing directly with one another for jobs, money and status.

But in addition to this, many women still want a good man for other reasons like a fulfilling relationship and children and, to some extent, they still have to compete with one another to attract the best mate. One key mechanism women traditionally used to compete for the best mate was to alter their appearance to attract a high-quality, resourceful male and one aspect of this is body shape. Dr Smith believes that this body competition mechanism has been distorted and activated unnecessarily within a culture that is ripe and ready to cultivate body dissatisfaction. If women with higher aspirations are exposed to other professional women who are slim and successful, it 'may lead some women to feel more ineffective and more dissatisfied with their bodies ... activating a default strategy of weight loss.'[57]

At a time when all the emphasis is on women being professionally successful and on removing barriers to that success, Smith's team have pointed to some inconvenient side effects. However, instead of seeing these findings as a threat to women's right to be professionally successful, and therefore politically incorrect, we should note the findings. An awareness of how our modern way of living may jar with what went before will enable us to cope with it better than we are at the moment.

The Flabs and the Flab-nots

Research is now finding a link between materialism and body image. Materialistic media encouraging women to aspire to the material 'good life' has 'a clear influence on women's body image'. And women who are already more materialistic have 'a further vulnerability factor for negative exposure effects in response to idealised, thin media models'.[58]

Body comparison and resulting body dissatisfaction are a form of social comparison – or keeping up with the Boneses – and have a lot in common with how the economy, or more precisely, social economics works. In the way that mass income inequality can lead to envy, dissatisfaction and social instability, so too body 'inequality' leads to widespread body dissatisfaction. If you or I have enough money and a reasonable standard of living, yet we are constantly exposed to many others who have far more money and a far better standard of living, we can experience *relative deprivation*: feeling deprived of something which we believe is achievable and to which we feel entitled. It is the gap between expectation and present actuality which, in the context of body dissatisfaction, is the flabs and the flab-nots. As is the case with having wealth rubbed in your face, so raising aspirations unrealistically, seeing ubiquitous body privilege generates dissatisfaction – relative body deprivation.

Body shape and comparison are more important than ever, and women's bodies have become more objectified and analysed by themselves than ever. Once your body is considered by you to be a separate entity to be adjusted and worked on, it is then commodified by the market place, which sells the possibility of owning a 'better' body shape. Put simply, the media, fashion industry, diet companies, food conglomerates (which own the diet companies), fitness industry and the pharmaceutical and cosmetic-surgery industries will make a far greater profit if you are dissatisfied with your body. High body esteem is bad for business.

Body dissatisfaction, on the other hand, is good for handbag and shoe sales. A New Zealand and Canadian research team found that the more insecure women feel when they see attractive female models, the more shoes and handbags they tended to own. It's thought that 'accessorizing becomes particularly appealing because it helps increase physical attractiveness without drawing attention to one's figure'.[59]

There is, however, one industry that may want to think twice about making women feel bad about their bodies. The medical and science journal *Appetite* published the study 'The effect of images of thin and overweight body shapes on women's ambivalence towards chocolate'. And the news isn't good for Cadbury's, Hershey's or Lindt. The scientists began by establishing that:

'Many women experience ambivalent orientations towards chocolate, both craving for it and having concerns about eating it', before going on to investigate 'the effect of viewing thin and overweight images of models in chocolate advertisements' on said ambivalence. Women were exposed to chocolate advertisements using either a thin model or an overweight model. Those who saw the adverts with thin models 'had increased avoidance, approach and guilt scores', while those who saw the adverts with overweight models 'had decreased approach and guilt scores, with no change in avoidance'.[60]

And speaking of guilt, it's now been found to be an emotion that can make you feel fatter than you really are. In a new series of studies, 'The Weight of a Guilty Conscience: Subjective Body Weight as an Embodiment of Guilt', researchers at Princeton discovered evidence that the emotional experience of guilt can literally become 'embodied' and affect your judgment of your weight. People prompted to experience guilt-inducing memories 'reported higher than average subjective body weight' regardless of their physical weight. They also found that 'immoral acts led to reports of increased subjective body weight.' But in case you're thinking of using this to go on a high-morality diet, the scientists have already been there, finding that 'unethical acts made participants feel heavier, but ethical acts did not make participants feel lighter'.[61]

So continuing the guilt theme, is there now enough evidence to find the media guilty, at the very least, for aiding and abetting our body dissatisfaction?

Two

Know Your Wiggle Room

When I think of body dissatisfaction the counterpart could, I suppose, be described as body aspiration: an underlying – or not so underlying – yearning for a different body.

In many ways it seems akin to a low-level yet ever-present unrequited love: you've met someone you're infatuated with, and after plenty of sex and good times you start to enquire, 'Where is this going? Don't worry, you can be honest with me.' And he is whispering, in maybe not so many words, in between kisses, 'Why rush things? I'm really happy with things the way they are.'

Ultimately, you want to hear the right noises about commitment and perhaps children. He wants to drink the milk without buying the cow. When asked directly 'Are we going to get married?' he dithers, so you cut to the chase with an erectile dysfunction-inducing query, such as, 'Do you love me?' He averts his gaze uncomfortably and, after a soul-searching pause, replies: 'No'. Wrong answer.

You end the relationship. But late one night, after reading

one of those *Fifty Shades of Grey*-type books or, worse yet, playing that tear-jerking Lady Antebellum song, 'Need You Now', you pick up the phone and enjoy a night of rapprochement. But nothing has changed fundamentally; it's just a nocturnal dalliance. The next day you call your best friend for advice which she offers without hesitation: 'He told you he doesn't love you. Says he'll never marry you or have children with you. Should I make an appointment for a hearing test?'

You take her point, hide the Lady Antebellum CD and put on Gotye's 'Somebody That I Used to Know' instead, realising that yours is a case of unrequited love for a man and a relationship that is unattainable.

There are parallels with trying unsuccessfully to have an unrealistic body size or shape. Although through diets and fat-burning classes you may enter an on/off flirtation with the dress size or body shape you want, in the long-term you may not be able to have the body you want to spend the rest of your life with.

A reality check on what is possible is a good factual point from which to start confronting body dissatisfaction. Any type of dissatisfaction involves the gap between what we want and believe is possible, versus what *is* possible. In trying to come to terms with many difficult things, understanding that gap and acknowledging the realities and limitations of actually being able to change the situation are likely to prevent or reduce our dissatisfaction.

If body dissatisfaction is more about 'feeling fat', irrespective of how fat you may or may not actually be, then we really need some universal science-based yardsticks against which to make our judgments. We'll come back to these yardsticks a bit later, but first, let's look at what actually determines our body shape, size and weight, to what extent we can change this – and, if we can, whether such changes are long-lasting.

You *Aren't* What You Eat

It is in the interests of various interests – namely the food, diet and fashion industries – that we believe our appearance can be bought. Our shape, we are encouraged to believe, is in our hands and our misshape is the result of slovenliness. Pear-shaped woman is more likely to be seen as having eaten her way to that shape, helped along by her fondness for spending time reclining on the sofa. Svelte woman on the other hand may be credited with greater self-discipline in the face of Ben & Jerry's and a preference for body-pump classes over sleeping. But when we stop and think about it, we all know people who can eat what and when they want and may prefer the elevator to the stairs, the sofa to the Zumba class, yet who seem relatively immune to gaining weight.

Genes vs jeans

While it may benefit the food, diet and fashion industries to depict your shape, weight and body composition as the product of what you do or don't do, this ignores an inconvenient and unprofitable truth. The places where you accumulate fat – that is, your pattern of body-fat distribution – and the ease with which you accumulate it are influenced by the genes you inherit. This explains why two women leading exactly the same lifestyle, eating the same things and taking the same amount of exercise may still end up with very different rear ends, accumulating different amounts of body fat and/or different patterns of distribution.

We inherit a blend of genes from our mother and father. We can be unlucky and get the worst possible combination from both parents or be fortunate and get the best.

For example, in a study published in the journal *Cell Metabolism*, UCLA researchers gave more than 100 different genetic strains of mice a normal diet for eight weeks, followed by a high-fat, high-sugar diet for another eight weeks. Even though all of the mice were eating the exact same diets, their weight gain varied greatly. The high-fat diet caused no change in body-fat percentage for some mice, while this increased by a whopping 600 per cent in others. Those differences were largely attributed to genetics. The scientists identified and compared eleven genetic regions associated with obesity and fat gain in the mice, several of which overlap with genes linked to obesity in humans.[1]

The UCLA researchers believe obesity to be 'a highly heritable disease driven by complex interactions between genetic and environmental factors'. The principal investigator said, 'If people consume a high-fat diet, the response will be predominantly determined by genetics, but whether you choose to eat a high-fat diet in the first place is largely environmental.'[2] In other words, we live unnaturally in a food-laden, 'obesogenic' environment, and if we have inherited the genes for easier fat gain – and are surrounded by an array of tempting overly available fattening foods – we will gain more body fat. Searching for a purely genetic explanation of excess weight gain in our world of abundance is misleading since any possible genetic control can be widely overshadowed by the effect of the environment.

Foetal programming and epigenetics

How much and what a mother eats before and during her pregnancy and the stress she experiences during pregnancy are now thought to play an important role in programming the future body shape and weight of the embryo and then foetus. A team at the University of California has outlined the 'Fetal Programming of Body Composition, Obesity, and Metabolic Function: The Role of Intrauterine Stress and Stress Biology', adding a vital, yet little-known dimension to our understanding of the origins of our body shape and size.[3] And as is already known, gaining excessive weight while you're pregnant increases the risk of your child becoming obese long after you give birth, from childhood right through to their adult years, even when you take into consideration other contributory fattening factors.[4]

Meanwhile, in mice they've found that pig-outs in pregnancy can increase the body size of offspring two generations later.[5]

Bon appetite

Our appetite traits, for example our responsiveness to food and how easily we're satisfied with the amount we're eating, is, from early infancy, strongly influenced by our genes.[6] People who carry two copies of a variant form of a particular gene are more likely to feel hungry soon after eating a meal and are biologically programmed to eat more. What's more, brain scans revealed that this changes the way in which the brain reacts to food and the appetite-stimulating hormone ghrelin, and can involve the brain's pleasure/reward centre that normally responds to alcohol and recreational drugs. The multinational team studying this added, 'Not only do these people have higher ghrelin levels and therefore feel hungrier, their brains respond differently to ghrelin and to pictures of food – it's a double hit.'[7]

About one in every six people carries two copies of this FTO gene variant and is 70 per cent more likely to become obese than those who carry other versions of it. Although the way and amount we eat has been viewed as complex, cultural and emotional in its causes, willpower is not enough to explain resistance to pigging out or losing weight. Controlling your appetite and weight is not merely a case of 'personal choice'.

NEAT

Non-exercise activity thermogenesis (NEAT) is the calories we burn for everything we do that is not sleeping, eating or physical exercise – so anything from walking to work and typing to gardening and fidgeting. NEAT could be an important factor in how we maintain/lose/gain weight. Even such calorie-burning fidgetiness is found to be 'primarily under genetic control'.[8]

Our shape-determining genes can be stubborn. Even disciplined dieters often find it difficult to lose weight or regain weight they've lost. Many researchers believe this is because each of us has a baseline weight – a genetically influenced 'set point' like a thermostat where our bodies naturally hover. If we reduce more than 10 per cent below our set point, our bodies will react and try to make up for it, and the more weight we lose, the harder our bodies work to compensate. We may become hungrier and our metabolism becomes more efficient at hanging on to those calories we eat.[9]

This isn't a reason for despair, but a way of understanding our situation, some of which simply is not fully under our control and, therefore, not necessarily our 'fault'.

Location, Location, Location

Few people are unhappy solely with their weight; body dissatisfaction is just as much – or more – about dissatisfaction with the various locations in which our body fat manages to luxuriate. We're displeased with our body-fat distribution, referred to by fat-researching scientists as human-fat topography. And the shipping terminology goes further: after the fat is distributed, the places where it is stored are referred to as fat 'depots'. But as is the case with the amount of fat we have and the ease with which we gain or lose it, its distribution – our shape – is also influenced by our inherited genes.

Body fat is a many and varied thing. As the German fat scientist Professor Manfred J. Müller puts it, our fat 'is heterogeneous with respect to location, amount present, metabolic functions, and response to weight changes'. He's called for 'a search for regulation of individual [fat] depots'.[10] Arnold Schwarzenegger's analysis – 'It's simple: if it jiggles, it's fat' – seems quaint in comparison.

But what drives fat distribution? Female sex hormones cause fat to be stored in the buttocks, thighs and hips. This 'gluteofemoral' pattern is what gives women their highly recognisable shape; it is subcutaneous fat, found just below the skin. Despite being almost universally loathed by its owners, this gluteofemoral fat may actually protect your health; yet fashion editors and the diet industry will not be going out of their way to tell you that scientists at Oxford University's Centre for Diabetes, Endocrinology and Metabolism have found 'a specific protective role of gluteofemoral body fat'. They believe this increased gluteofemoral fat may ensure women have healthier levels of fats and sugar in their bloodstream, as well as a reduction in their risk of cardiovascular disease, diabetes and stroke. They actively sing this fat's praises: 'This underlines gluteofemoral fat's role as a determinant of health.'[11]

Pear-shaped people, men as well as women, seem to be less prone to the harmful consequences of moderate obesity than those who are apple-shaped (see below). This may be because fat around the hips is less likely to be mobilised during stress; therefore, it remains in the hips and does not enter the bloodstream where it can become deposited in the walls of blood vessels. When women reach menopause and the oestrogen produced by ovaries declines, fat migrates from their buttocks, hips and thighs to their waists; later, fat is stored in the belly.

Android fat distribution is the distribution of fat tissue mainly around our trunk and upper body, in areas such as the stomach, chest, shoulder and nape of the neck. This pattern may lead to an 'apple-shaped' or central obesity, and is more common in men than in women. The intra-abdominal fat, is located inside the abdominal cavity, packed between the organs, and excessive amounts are also linked to type-2 diabetes, insulin resistance, inflammatory and other obesity-related diseases.

Body-fat distribution: android (apple-shaped) and gynoid (pear-shaped)

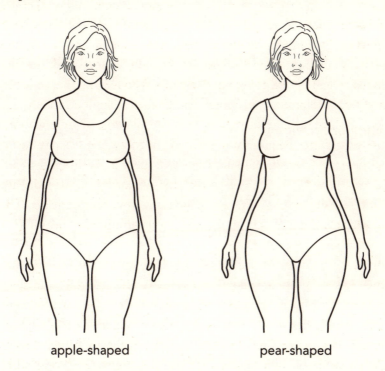

apple-shaped   pear-shaped

Body fat is an active part of your endocrine (hormone) system, providing feedback for hunger and diet to your brain. So what you do to your body fat – for example, dieting or starving it – can change the way it behaves and how it grows.

Returning to the issue of inheriting your body-fat distribution, researchers are reporting 'sex-specific genetic effects' on how your fat is distributed around your waist, hips and thighs.[12] When tracking the 'stability of subcutaneous fat distribution' all the way from early adolescence into young adulthood', geneticists found that genes played a highly significant role in how body-fat distribution changes over time and where it ends up by adulthood. Or as a study published in *Obesity Research* reassuringly puts it, 'Body fat and distribution ... are under extensive genetic control.'[13]

Your parents really do have a lot to answer for.[14]

And you may soon be able to blame your racial background too. Scientists at Northern Illinois University measured how much fat women of various ethnic backgrounds had in various parts of their bodies and reported 'a pattern of ethnic/race-related influence on regional fat deposition'.[15]

White or brown fat?

All fat is not equal. When we discuss and then condemn body fat we fail to show the right kind of colour-based discrimination between white and brown fat tissue.

The bulges on our body we deplore contain almost all white fat or white adipose tissue. However, we also harbour brown fat or brown adipose tissue (BAT), and brown fat cells have a great capacity to burn white fat and are also known to powerfully counteract obesity in rodents. It has also been shown that some forms of obesity in mice are linked to an inherited lack of brown fat. In short, it's thought that some of us may inherit more brown fat and/or our brown fat is more easily activated to burn our white body fat, which may keep us slimmer with little effort.[16]

Personality

Fat distribution isn't the only aspect of weight or shape we may inherit, nor is it the only predisposing influence on them. Studies suggest pretty convincingly that there are aspects of our temperament and character that may be associated with obesity and that neuropsychological factors play an important role in causing it.

When researchers assess our 'temperament and character' by measuring dimensions of personality in those of us who are lean vs those of us who are not so lean they find that obese people score higher in 'novelty-seeking', significantly lower in persistence and in self-directedness. Novelty-seeking is not only strongly linked with obesity, but also with difficulty in losing weight.[17]

A major study by researchers at the National Institutes of Health, examining 50 years of data on body fat, waist and hip circumference and personality traits refined and reinforced this link. It was the first to examine whether personality is linked with fluctuations in weight over time. People were assessed on major personality traits, along with many subcategories of these traits. Among other things, they found that impulsivity related to the novelty-seeking found in the study above was the strongest predictor of obesity: 'Previous research has found that impulsive individuals are prone to binge eating and alcohol consumption,' the lead researcher said. 'These behavioral patterns may contribute to weight gain over time.' In addition to greater weight gain among impulsive people, those who enjoy taking risks and those who are antagonistic (especially those who are cynical, competitive and aggressive) are more likely to accrue more body fat. Over the longer term, people with personality traits of high neuroticism and low conscientiousness were more likely to go through cycles of gaining and losing weight throughout their lives.[18]

31

This is not to say that there is a 'fat personality type'. Rather, it may be that some particularly high or low scores on certain dimensions of temperament or character – and the corresponding neurobiological patterns – may, together with other genetic and environmental factors, contribute to a predisposition for gaining body fat or for reaching our full potential for becoming obese.

Bringing up the rear

Although a mother's influence on her daughter's body image will be discussed later in Chapter 11, 'In Our Own Image', there is anecdotal evidence that grown women may continue to be influenced by their mother's current body image and actual body weight and shape. Therapists who have female patients with body-image problems or disordered eating may hear them talk about feelings and anxieties regarding their mothers' bodies: grown women who have never been overweight can become worried about gaining body fat because they're concerned about looking like their larger mothers; or, women who are naturally thin, but not as slender as their mothers can end up feeling inadequate. Some therapists mention competition between mothers and daughters which can manifest in terms of weight and shape because so much cultural emphasis is placed on body appearance.

Hormones: harmony and hell

Quite aside from everything mentioned above, there's the issue of the hormones in your life. Much is written about this at the popular end of the publishing market – for example, *From Belly Fat to Belly Flat: How Your Hormones Are Adding Inches to Your Waist*.

To start with there's perimenopause, the stage of your life that begins several years before menopause, when the ovaries gradually begin to produce less oestrogen. It usually starts in a woman's forties, but can start in the thirties or even earlier and is related to increased weight and a change in fat distribution. A bigger waistline is more likely after menopause. As the charming gynaecologists at the University of Pisa sing it, 'Menopause is associated with an accelerated increase in body weight and body fat, with a prevalent central, android fat distribution.'[19]

In animal studies, oestrogen seems to help regulate body weight with animals tending to eat more and be less physically active when their oestrogen levels are lower. Lower oestrogen may also reduce our metabolic rate – the rate at which we burn calories – and this may happen in women when their oestrogen levels decline after menopause. On top of that, you are less likely to exercise and you also you lose muscle mass, which lowers your resting metabolism, making it easier to gain body fat. Your aerobic fitness also declines.

Reality Check

So going back to those yardsticks – if body dissatisfaction really is more about 'feeling fat' and/or misshapen, regardless of how we actually are, our society has to shift its source of information and self-judgment to a fair and accurate source based on heavily researched scientific criteria, originating far away from Hollywood and our own underlying assumptions and insecurities. Here are those yardsticks.

The scales of justice

There are important limitations in using our body weight as a measure of our health and fitness. Body weight is important, but it's best used in conjunction with other measures and some common sense. There is no one 'ideal' weight for all people of a particular height because each individual's healthiest weight depends on their bone structure, muscle mass, body fat and general body build. So how can you decide on what is a healthy weight for you, and know if you are overweight or obese?

A healthy body weight is more about the way the body functions, what it's made up of and wellbeing than any media-defined beauty standards. There are three tools which, when used together, can accurately determine whether or not our body weight is healthy. They are:

- **body mass index** (BMI), which takes into consideration our height and weight
- **body shape**, which takes into consideration body-fat distribution
- **percentage body fat,** which takes into consideration our total fat stores.

You can calculate these measurements using the tools in the Appendix (see p. 208).

Body mass index (BMI)

Judging ourselves solely on our body weight can be misleading and may cause unnecessary body dissatisfaction. BMI is a measurement used to determine our level of fat in the context of our weight and height; it does not take into account our bone structure, which can skew the results. The numbers are often used to determine whether we're obese or overweight.

BMI calculations may categorise big-boned or muscular people as obese, notes the Harvard School of Public Health. Bone and muscle are denser than fat, making people with denser bones and more muscle weigh more. So an athlete with high bone density and more developed muscles may have a high

BMI, but not be medically overweight or obese. On the other hand, having a lower bone density, particularly osteoporosis, is strongly associated with a lower weight and body mass index. Few of us add muscle and bone after our early twenties, so nearly all the extra weight we put on is fat.[20]

Body shape

Once you know your BMI, and have a general idea of your level of body fatness, there's the question of where your body fat is located. This is where the android/gynoid types of body-fat distribution (apple vs pear shape) discussed above come into the equation. In short, if you carry the bulk of your body fat above your hips (mainly in your abdomen), you have an apple shape. People who are apple shaped sometimes have a larger waist than hips and when they gain body fat, it tends to go directly to their stomach. People who carry the bulk of their weight in their extremities (hips, thighs and buttocks) are described as having a pear shape; they generally have larger hips than waist.

Whether you are an apple or a pear is less important unless you are overweight according to your BMI. If you are overweight or obese, having an apple shape puts you at much higher risk for heart disease, type-2 diabetes, hypertension and several types of cancer. For those who naturally become apple shaped with weight gain, it is critically important that a healthy body weight be maintained.

You can easily gauge whether you are an apple or pear shape or perhaps a hybrid fruit, by calculating your waist-to-hip ratio (see p. 212).

Percentage body fat

In order to further identify women who appear to have a normal BMI, but have actually been 'misclassified' because they are made up of too much body fat, 'fat-ologists' have developed a number of tools to measure *how much* of our body is made up of fat i.e. our 'adiposity'. Techniques such as hydrodensito-metry (underwater weighing), DEXA (dual energy X-ray absorptiometry) or MRI fat scans are expensive and usually available only in research centres or hospitals. So for most people the best method is 'pinch-an-inch' anthropometry (skin-fold thickness measures), which should be done by your local nurse, doctor or other practitioner who is trained and used to carrying out these measurements. If you are determined to do it yourself, you can buy hand-held skin calipers online and follow the instructions to measure skinfold thickness at various body locations (three to seven test sites are common). A calculation is then used to derive a body fat percentage based on the sum of the numbers. The accuracy is not as high as the high-tech methods above; however, skinfold measurements are easy to establish, inexpensive and convenient.

Bioelectric impedance analysis (BIA) is considered more accurate than calipers. BIA equipment sends a small, impercep-tible, safe electric current through the body, measuring the resistance. The current faces more resistance passing through body fat than it does passing through lean body mass and water. BIA equipment is available at many health clubs and gyms or online.[21]

This area of medicine is still undecided in terms of exactly how much fat is or isn't a risk. However, some researchers now believe that women who fall within the normal range for BMI (18.5–24.9), yet are made up of more than 30 per cent body fat are at greater health risk.[22] Once you have a good estimate of your percentage body fat, check your numbers against the table in the Appendix (see p. 211).

'Fit and toned'?

The London 2012 Olympics were accompanied by plenty of rhetoric. Among the surplus of hyperbole were assured assertions about gold medallists being particularly important to girls and women as 'strong female role models'. However, researchers at Brunel University, School of Sport and Education are concerned about the negative effects on young women of this hijacking and distortion of the role of female gold medallists. The ongoing research project CelebYouth is examining how 'celebrity is impacting negatively on young people's aspirations'. Faculty member Heather Mendick spotted the process in action, describing how journalists and social commentators celebrated the 'real' role models that the Olympics offered girls and young women. Unlike the many excellent accomplished role models girls have had for decades, these were 'authentic', 'empowering' and 'inspiring' figures for young female audiences. Girlguiding UK were so inspired they launched their 'Real Role Models' campaign. Newspapers in most countries glorified women competitors' six-packs and non-existent hips along with bicep and deltoid muscle definition that put most men to shame. These gold medallists were portrayed as being at the apex of what it means to be being 'fit and toned'.

The average female heptathlete will have somewhere between 10 and 14 per cent body fat – half that of normal women. Furthermore, female Olympic athletes may actually be poor role models for female body image. There is a recognised complication in female athletes involving a combination – or 'triad' – of insufficient nutrition, cessation of menstruation and bone weakness and fractures, due to insufficient hormone levels. They often have eating disorders, some of which do not fit into the usual anorexia/bulimia categories, and are called

Eating Disorders Not Otherwise Specified (EDNOS). Few people are aware that the International Olympic Committee Medical Commission Working Group Women in Sport are so concerned that they have published a 'Position Stand [on] a cascade of events labelled the Female Athlete Triad', including the interrelated problems of disordered eating, complete absence of or infrequent menstruation (amenorrhoea) and osteoporosis.[23]

Scientists at the University of Wisconsin School of Medicine and Public Health, who strangely enough don't work for the cosmetics, media or fashion industries, are now reporting that 'mounting evidence demonstrates that the triad is present in the high-school population'.[24] In an earlier study they found that 26.9 per cent of female athletes had disordered eating and menstrual dysfunction and 10.2 per cent had disordered eating and low bone density. And the scientists found that 'the triad is also present in normal active females' and that prevention of one or more of its components 'should be geared towards all physically active girls and young women'.[25]

In a recent study of long-term consequences of the female athlete triad researchers followed up women who were diagnosed with the syndrome as adolescents and young adults back in the 1990s and who are now in their thirties and forties and found that negative long-term effects 'such as low bone-mineral density are now starting to manifest'.[26]

Despite the beauty adverts featuring the very same 'fit-and-toned' female Olympic stars, another study overturns widely held popular assumptions: 'Female athletes prove to have higher body dissatisfaction on themselves compared to female non-athletes', along with a troubled relationship with food.[27] Yet female celebrity competitors appeared as idealised role models in beauty adverts throughout and beyond the Olympics. In the mistaken belief that the images of lean-and-mean, low-fat, ripped bodies of female medallists are just the healthy anti-dote we need to counteract the size-zero culture of stick-thin models, journalists in major national newspapers hailed these bodies as superb examples of what girls and women *should* now venerate. A glowing column in the *Observer* said: 'Buoyed up by the life-affirming images of lean and muscular British female athletes ... Now, after London 2012, all women can value their bodies and play to their strengths ... we have a new generation of role models to aspire to, whose bodies are revered for their physical abilities and not just their aesthetic qualities.' It was all about looks and performance with no knowledge of real female health or any of the studies mentioned above. Away from the catwalk, even intelligent, considered discussion about bodies and health is steered, not by health experts, but by the media and the images the media see within the media and then comment on.

We've accepted a blanket prescription that 'thin is healthy' and nod in agreement when we hear media-derived phrases such as 'fit and toned'. But the definition of these throwaway phrases has been just as distorted as the body image of most women. Research and real life now make it clear that thin is by no means necessarily healthy and that being pear-shaped and having hip and thigh fat is often extremely healthy (and sexually attractive too). It's very apparent that the yardstick for gauging body image has to be wrenched back from the food, diet and fashion industries, the media ... and our own common beliefs. And this, in turn, has to be accompanied by new ground rules about who is to be trusted when discussing dress size, body-fat distribution, body size and weight. Next time you 'feel fat', let the fat experts – not the fashion experts or media commentators – carry out a reality check on your self-judgments.

Piling On the £ounds

A gargantuan market is benefiting from today's normative discontent. Despite an appalling 95 per cent failure rate in helping people keep their weight off, the diet industry (often described as the most successful failed business in the world) continues to grow fat and is currently valued at $61 billion in the US alone and £1 billion in the UK.

Any diet can enable you to lose weight, but keeping it off has been a spectacular failure. To this end, diets don't work; but from deflab to reflab and back, those running the repeat customer diet industry are always in work. Dieting is not merely an extension of a makeover. Dieting – a sudden temporary reduction in calories to lose weight – has recently been found to be a 'major medical event', causing significant metabolic, neuroendocrine and epigenetic alterations in those who attempt to diet, in some cases paradoxically leading to disease. Intermittent ('yo-yo') dieting increasingly practised in response to body dissatisfaction could end up reprogramming your food preferences, promoting the 'compulsive selection' of fatty, sugary unhealthy food and the undereating of healthy foods, and may be accompanied by 'a withdrawal-like state seen in drug dependence'.[28] This eating pattern leads to a vicious circle. The more you do it, the more likely it is that you will do it again – good for the diet companies, but very bad for your size, shape, health and life expectancy. Weight cycling (losing and then regaining a small amount of weight), averaging only 2.5kg over two-year periods among people who are normal weight is strongly linked to 'a higher risk of cardiovascular disease and death'.[29] For more on dieting, see Chapter 12, 'Downsizing'.

Ironically, research now finds that improving body image may actually enhance the effectiveness of weight-loss programmes that are based on healthy eating and physical activity. The authors go on to say, 'From this we believe that learning to relate to your body in healthier ways is an important aspect of maintaining weight loss and should be addressed in every weight-control programme.'[30]

Obesogenic Environment

As a young child, I, like many other children often heard the refrain, 'Finish your dinner; just think of all those poor, starving children in China!' Yet when I visit China nowadays, the children there are beginning to resemble Americans in their physique. Travelling to many foreign countries has made me privy to another form of reality check, enabling me to answer the simple question: do people in countries with inexpensive high-calorie, highly processed foods become fat? Absolutely. An obesity epidemic has replaced the spectre of starvation in many 'developing' countries to such an extent that it's described by public health professionals as a 'wicked problem'. As nations grow economically, traditional diets are supplanted by cheap, imported and obesogenic foods.

For instance, Tonga's climate is idyllic and it has an abundance of its own natural, healthy food: fish, pigs, sweet potatoes and mangoes. Yet I saw young people embracing many of the same junk foods we see here in the West, and although body confidence isn't the problem there that it is in the West, obesity is: the prevalence of obesity among women in Tonga now is twice that of American women.

It is not merely a question of self-discipline and personal choice: what you are surrounded by and tempted with has a direct effect on your body size, weight and shape – so much so that in dealing with this 'wicked problem', the Harvard College

Global Health Review states the 'devastating obesity epidemic ... is directly caused by social and political choices' and recommends 'that governments take actions to directly alter the obesogenic environment'.[31] Professors from the Harvard School of Public Health and the World Health Organization published a key paper in the *Lancet* which also puts paid to the idea that *you* are the sole architect of your own body shape: 'Governments are the most important actors in reversing the obesity epidemic.'[32]

Julie Guthman at the University of California, is concerned at how even the most seemingly liberal minds among students in a very liberal part of America seem to have embraced the idea that it's the individual who determines his own body fat, as opposed to the obesogenic environment. Guthman's paper 'Teaching the Politics of Obesity: Insights into Neoliberal Embodiment and Contemporary Biopolitics', steps back from the specific causes of excess body fat: 'Student responses demonstrate how obesity talk reflects and reinforces neoliberal rationalities of self-governance, particularly those that couple bodily control and deservingness and see fatness as weakening the health of the body politic.' In short, through believing in democratic notions of free will and choice, young people had unknowingly discounted the genetic, biological and environment interactions just described.[33]

So we have to remind ourselves that much of our battle of the bulge is the result of the supply of calorie-rich food in our culture. A short while ago, not many people had ready access to a lot of food, so only those with an extremely high susceptibility to weight gain became overweight. Today, for just a few pounds, even someone with genes predisposing them to be more slender can buy enough food to supersize themselves. We are living in a world for which our genes just weren't designed.

This is by no means a fat sentence. But what it does mean is that given our genetic disposition and the environment we live in, we can only expect so much of ourselves. While we may not be able to change being apple-shaped, it's certainly well within our power to be the healthiest, fittest apple possible. Armed with knowledge about body size, shape and composition, our family background and genetic predispositions, and prior success (or lack of it) in trying to create a lasting change to our body weight, size and shape, we can arrive at a far healthier and happier place in future. Confronting body dissatisfaction requires knowing our wiggle room. And no one person's wiggle room is the same as someone else's.

Three

A Source of Thinspiration

Comparison is the thief of joy.
Theodore Roosevelt

Given the growing concern about the effect of media images of the great and the slender on our body satisfaction, an obvious question comes to mind: if we never saw images of slim, beautiful people, would we be more satisfied with our own bodies? Is body image literally a case of out of sight, out of mind?

Two studies on blind women support the adage that what the eye doesn't see, the heart doesn't grieve over, and also that ignorance really can be bliss. The first – 'Body image dissatisfaction and eating attitudes in visually impaired women' – reported that women who are born blind 'had lower body dissatisfaction scores and more positive eating attitudes compared to women blinded later in life and sighted women, the latter having the highest body dissatisfaction scores and the most negative eating attitudes'.[1] Ten years later, a second study – 'Body image and restrained eating in blind and sighted women' – found the same: 'Blind women were more satisfied with their body and dieted less than sighted women.' The researchers pointed to an obvious suspect: 'the importance of visual exposure to the media's thin ideal'.[2]

Another way of looking at this is to study 'media-naive' cultures that are exposed to TV images for the first time, to see if there are any changes in female body image and behaviour.

Tonga

Half a world away, I arrive in Tonga, on the International Date Line, where day and night are the absolute opposite of the time zone I left behind, and so are the body politics. Tongans look like goddesses and warriors: they are big, natural people. The women have names like Fi and Sessie. They have big, feminine hips and walk with a noticeable absence of self-consciousness, which is also apparent in their lack of concern about their body shape and size. The national beauty contest is a potpourri of full-figured, chunky contestants, and the winner is big.

When I boarded a tiny sixteen-seat aeroplane to fly between islands, the women, most of them heavier than me, showed no embarrassment at being publicly weighed with their baggage on an enormous set of scales for all to see. Imagine having *your* weight displayed for all to see at Heathrow or JFK airport?

But the arrival of American DVDs in the year 2000 changed their bodies and their language. The new generation of girls are suddenly showing signs of change in a Westerly direction. They tell me they want to be slimmer like the women they see on the global screen. A more global gait and cadence is starting to appear among the younger women.

Fiji

About 500 miles to the west, in the Fijian islands, the effects of television on a foreign culture are truly laid bare. Television has gone beyond changing body language to causing actual bodily changes.

In a landmark study, a multidisciplinary team from Harvard Medical School travelled to Fiji to evaluate the impact of the introduction of television on body satisfaction and disordered eating in adolescent girls. In Fiji, the ideal body for females was always very full, while 'going thin' – as Fijians refer to weight loss – was cause for concern, not admiration. Dieting was rare.

In 1995, however, television arrived and within three years everything changed. The percentage of girls with pathologically high scores on a test for disordered eating more than doubled from 12.7 per cent to 29.2 per cent and three-quarters of the study population reported that they felt 'too big or fat'. Dieting among teenagers who started to watch television increased dramatically to include two in every three girls, and the rate of self-induced vomiting to control weight, which had previously been rated as non-existent, leaped to 11.3 per cent of that population. The girls openly cited thin female characters in American programmes as inspirations for changing their bodies. Comments included: 'I feel fat', 'I just admire them', 'I want their body', 'I want their size'.

The researchers describe the 'dramatic increase' in disordered eating: 'The impact of television appears especially profound … Western media imagery may have a profoundly negative impact upon body image and disordered eating attitudes and behaviours, even in traditional societies in which eating disorders have been thought to be rare.'[3]

46

Shangri-la

For centuries, Bhutan remained in self-imposed isolation from outside influences, and it is its undiluted culture that attracts the few tourists who have been allowed in since it cautiously opened its doors forty years ago. The King of Bhutan emphasises the importance of retaining cultural integrity and promoting national identity, traditional values and the concept of One Nation, One People. Most important is the ideal of gross national happiness. If there was a Shangri-la, this was truly it.

However, in June 1999 Bhutan became the last nation on earth to introduce television and I was there as the cultural experiment unfolded. Bhutan's political and geographical isolation, coupled with the suddenness with which its people were been exposed to forty-six cable channels, made it the perfect social laboratory.

The Bhutan Broadcasting Service (BBS) provides 'a local educational and cultural service', consisting of an hour a day of amateur-quality religious footage directly from a Buddhist temple. I managed to see some of it and marvelled at how quaint and wholesome it seemed. During my visit to Bhutan, the Ministry of Health held a small conference attended by the country's main health officials, and it happened to be in the dining room of the small hotel I was staying in. I was invited to the conference dinner, which was to be followed by traditional dancing.

During the conference, I talked to a number of doctors about the differences in health concerns between Bhutan and Britain and the United States. There was, for example, discussion and great concern about the link between the Bhutanese penchant for eating raw chillies and the prevalence of stomach cancer. I reciprocated by talking of the mounting Western health issues of obesity, eating disorders, stress-related diseases and depression, and caused raised eyebrows when I elaborated on new forms of elective surgery such as liposuction and the 'trout pout', before moving embarrassingly on to penis enlargement and the lunchtime boob job. I was, however, intrigued by their view of how the introduction of television might affect the health, wellbeing and gross national happiness of Bhutan. They didn't seem particularly concerned about the effects. In fact, I sensed an innocent, but enormous, gap in their comprehension of what television would do, not only to their culture, but to the health of the nation as well. It seemed that the government had thought that while real tourists in the flesh would lead to irreversible changes in their country, ephemeral electronic images delivered from afar didn't feature very highly as either a cultural or a health issue. I said to them, 'Don't you realise what Western television will do? Do you have any idea how influential it is?' They listened politely, but I honestly don't believe they understood my point.

Shortly after I returned home, I was shocked to read that Bhutan was experiencing its first crime wave – murder, fraud and drug offences. While it was television-free, this country had never experienced serious law-breaking. Bhutanese academics conducted an impact study and reported that television has caused 'dramatic changes': increasing crime, corruption, an uncontrolled desire for Western products and dramatically changing attitudes to relationships – including those between women and their own bodies. One third of girls suddenly wanted to look more American (whiter skin, blonde hair). The Minister of Health and Education, Sangay Ngedup, was one of the only members of the government willing to openly express his concerns about television. 'You can never predict the impact of things like TV ...' Nowadays however, you can.

And it now seems that no culture is immune to these effects on body image.

Body Image of Immigrants

Instead of observing what happens when the slender screen images come to your culture, other scientists stay put and watch what happens when you enter a culture which is already awash with slim images and cultural values to match. Psychologists at University of California, Berkeley found that young 'Asian-American' (i.e. Chinese, Japanese, Korean) women were not immune to the negative effects of media exposure on their body satisfaction and 'may be employing unhealthy weight-control behaviors, and may be prone to developing eating disorders, at rates similar to European American young adult females'. They emphasised the importance of how the Asian-American women may internalise 'the thin ideal', learning values and attitudes about female body size and shape that are incorporated within themselves and set them up for body dissatisfaction.[4] Similarly, studies of young Mexican-American women looked at two distinct types of body dissatisfaction: global evaluations of entire weight and shape and 'site-specific evaluations' (i.e. thighs or calves). And their conclusion wasn't very patriotic-sounding: 'The relationships between acculturation toward dominant U.S. culture and both types of body dissatisfaction were found to be fully mediated by internalization of U.S. standards of female beauty.'[5]

Permarexic People

Convinced by the overwhelming evidence that images can have powerful effects on the health of girls and women, the Israeli government has become the first to outlaw fashion models with a body mass index (BMI) of below 18.5 (the minimum 'normal' weight) from the catwalk, as well as from photo shoots and advertising campaigns. It also bans the use of models who 'appear underweight', meaning advertisers are not allowed to make a model's body look thinner than it really is using air-brushing. Brands which digitally alter photographs to trim away unwanted weight from models will have to clearly mark the resulting images to indicate that they have been manipulated. Following a rise in eating disorders in Israeli society, par-ticularly among young girls, the bill was co-drafted by Dr Rachel Adatto a legislator and physician, who said underweight models, 'can no longer serve as role models for innocent young people who adopt and copy the illusion of thinness'.[6]

But while most concern has surrounded thin fashion models, greater risk may lie in the more everyday ambient images of 'permarexic' – visibly unhealthily thin – television presenters, actresses and newsreaders, who form the backdrop to the visual lives of girls and women. For example, a few years ago, when doing research for a biology paper I was writing, I tried to assess the body sizes and fat distribution of female children's BBC TV presenters and found at that time that not a single one approached an average body weight with normal fat distribution. Even the prime-time evening female news anchors appeared thin or permarexic. And this streamlined look seems to have become an international franchise. In most countries I've visited, the picture on the screen is a variation on the same theme: collar bones, lollipop heads and the veneer of merely being 'fit and toned' because they 'work out' and build 'healthy muscle'.

When I wrote this very chapter I was in Santiago de Compostela, northern Spain. Every morning in the hotel restau-rant I looked at a large silent TV screen with twenty-four-hour news. Alongside actual film of Spain's worst train tragedy, killing eighty people which happened just outside of town, or news footage showing the bodies of freshly killed Egyptians being laid side by side, the all-female news anchors were, without exception, extremely slender, as were the female reporters covering stories on the ground. My limited ability to translate the Spanish-language teletext running along the bottom of the screen compounded by a lack of sound provided an acute insight into the aesthetic dimension, the real subtext of who is seen to be knowing, competent, glamorous and in charge on the news screen.

Yet any serious correlation between visual media and the rise of body dissatisfaction and eating disorders was until recently largely dismissed. We were told by media execs that 'the images merely reflect what women think looks good and so why not give them what they obviously prefer?' And until now, so-called 'body politics' has been a cultural and psychological debate, confined to feminists and eating-disorder therapists, and blaming the visual media was deemed too simplistic.

However, new research shows there is a much stronger link between visual media, body dissatisfaction and eating disorders.

But how can media actually change our self-worth?

From photo to frump

Unlike the studies above of cultures or groups that are exposed to slim, 'beautiful' media images over a period of time, laboratory-based studies have tried to see if there are immediate effects on body dissatisfaction and eating-disorder symptoms, with mixed results, probably due to the short-term nature of the experiments. One recent analysis of thirty-three lab studies concluded: 'In summary, our meta-analysis clearly reveals that media exposure of the ideal physique results in small changes in eating-disorder symptoms, particularly with participants at high risk for developing an eating disorder ... Even though the impact of any one brief media exposure on mood and body image is small ...

over time, the effects of many such small changes may cumulate to actually elevate body image disturbance.'[7]

While attention has so far focused on the effects of *slim* female media physiques, new studies are examining the contemporary 'fit-and-toned' language of camouflage increasingly used to rebrand unhealthy images of women. An interesting study on 'The effect of viewing ultra-fit images on college women's body dissatisfaction' spotted the trend that 'modern ideals of female attractiveness include an extremely toned and fit appearance in addition to extreme thinness'. And when the experimenters exposed young women to this new breed of thin, 'fit-and-toned' image they found it produced an increase in body dissatisfaction.[8]

Yet many magazine editors and readers themselves often say that far from making them feel unhappy about their own bodies, seeing the idealised body images in women's magazines actually inspires them and makes them feel good. Indeed, a study from Ohio State University found that women 'who were exposed to thin-ideal messages for five days in a row reported increases in their body satisfaction'. But the reasons for this are interesting, as 'exposure to thin-ideal body images leads to more dieting behaviours, possibly more exercising and ultimately enhances body satisfaction most likely through these mediators. In other words, viewing magazine pages with thin body ideals appears to induce behaviour changes and, as a result, increases body satisfaction.' At this point, magazine execs may claim that it's a win–win process, whereby their readers are not only enjoying themselves and feeling better about their bodies after looking at other women's slimmer bodies, but they are inspired to 'go for it' and lead a healthier lifestyle. However, all is not rosy.

In the middle-term, exposure to such idealised body images may motivate women to engage in 'body-shaping behaviours'. By comparing yourself with others who are better off, even with stars and celebrities, you may aspire to greater success for yourself: a form of self-improvement motivation. Your resulting dietary action plan then enhances your body satisfaction, at least for the time being. And in the hope of a slimmer body, women may engage in exposure to idealised body messages, which encourage them to diet; then, after engaging in self-improvement behaviours like dieting, they feel better about their bodies. This, in turn, may lead women to consume more of these messages in order to maintain the dieting motivation. And so the cycle continues, as do the financial profits for the industries that provide the images and services.

However, much to the chagrin of the vast majority of dieters, dieting is known to result in long-term weight gain – you end up back in reflab. And if the lack of dieting success is attributed to oneself (i.e. your lack of self-control), you may well continue to attend to body-ideal images and messages, hoping to diet with more success in the future. Researchers highlight the paradox of women appearing to expose themselves voluntarily to messages that undermine their self-esteem in this way – and they certainly don't recommend it. 'Fighting a losing battle against body weight, fuelled by media exposure to unrealistic ideals, consumes too much of women's psychological and financial resources and hurts their physical and mental health.'[9]

And there are further nuances to the way women respond to slim images in the short term. Marketing researchers have pointed to 'defensive reactions to slim female images in advertising' and theorise that the effect on women differs based on how blatantly or subtly the idealised slim images are presented. When they are presented blatantly – unobscured, focusing clearly on the subjects' slender beauty – we may detect the ideal being rubbed in our faces; this elicits a defensive coping mechanism to fortify our own self-image as if to say, 'I see what you're trying to do here, and I'm not being duped by it'. As a result, a rise in self-esteem may actually be reported. But when the images are exposed subtly –

say, in the context of a product being advertised or as an after-thought – they operate under the radar without us realising and we end up feeling worse about ourselves.[10]

One team of psychologists believes that when our favourite slim celebrities are involved we tend to assume a likeness between ourselves and the people we admire. And so by a process called assimilation, we associate the positive feelings we have about Miley Cyrus or Jennifer Aniston, for example, with positive feelings about ourselves. The 'parasocial' (one-sided) relationship we establish with these slender celebs therefore protects us from feeling more dissatisfied with our own bodies. It was found that women who thought they shared a birthday with a slender model felt better about their bodies after seeing her photo than women who felt they had nothing common with the model. Similarly, women who were shown one of their favourite thin celebrities felt better about their own figures than when shown thin celebrities who they didn't like.[11] However, what a person says they feel at the time they're looking at their favourite celeb is not the same as the cumulative long-term effects.

If viewing idealised images of slender women may have a negative effect on your own body satisfaction and what you strive for in changing your own body shape and size, what happens if you are exposed to images of models of a typical healthy weight instead? Does it also work the other way? As I'm writing this, the Department of Psychology at the University of Massachusetts has published 'Body ideals in women after viewing images of typical and healthy-weight models', providing some encouraging answers: 'We found that after viewing images of healthy-weight models, women's body ideals were significantly larger than when the same women viewed images of very thin models. This effect was greatest in those women with the highest levels of baseline anxiety ... viewing healthy-weight models results in more healthy body ideals than those typically promoted through media.'[12]

Mad methods

Desperate body concerns have been known to result in bizarre measures. For example, in the early 1930s women were led to believe they could simply wash away their body fat. 'Slimming soaps' such as 'Fatoff', 'Fat-O-NO' and 'La-Mar Reducing Soap' had women diving into the bathtub. Then the 1960s spawned the 'Sleeping Beauty Diet', the logic being you simply can't eat while you're asleep. Devotees would heavily sedate themselves and sleep for days.[13]

Males vs females

As we'll see in Chapter 6, 'Manorexia', men too have body-image disorders and are affected by media images; however, it manifests itself in a different way and far less is known about men and body dissatisfaction and eating disorders. Women, on the other hand, have been studied extensively and it appears they are particularly vulnerable to the effects of idealised media images. The question is how do images actually have their effect on a woman's brain and mind?

Women appear neurologically predisposed to be highly susceptible to body dissatisfaction if the media environment is awash with endless images of slender women. Repeated exposure to images of thin women may alter brain function and increase a woman's propensity to develop eating disorders.

While the media enjoys politically charged – and often politically correct – debates and discussions about differences between men and women's brains and minds, most reasonable scientists believe that there are some general differences. Those previously worried that highlighting these could be used to diminish women's status should wake up to the fact that many of the differences under discussion could, in fact, be used to show women as more capable and better equipped to deal with modern demands than their counterpart – the so-called 'redundant male'.

Yet when it comes to body image, women are more likely to do themselves down, according to the study 'Exploring Body Comparison Tendencies: Women Are Self-Critical Whereas Men Are Self-Hopeful'. Women were found to rely on 'self-critical social comparison strategies associated with negative body esteem' while on the other hand 'men's comparison strategies and perfection beliefs were more self-hopeful'. Furthermore, women were most likely to compare themselves to someone with a 'better' body shape than them – an 'upward social comparison'.[14]

There are differences between men and women in both their overall and specific types of self-esteem, as well as the incidence of some psychiatric disorders related to self-esteem. This suggests that there are gender differences in the neural basis underlying self-esteem. In the first study to explore this, neuroscientists 'showed significantly different brain activity between males and females' with key brain regions in a woman 'more activated than males when her self-positivity is threatened'. The researchers believe these differences in brain activity related to self-esteem 'may explain female cognitive/behavioral traits; females tend to ruminate more often than males, which sometimes results in a prolonged negative effect'.[15]

Women's brains are also highly attuned to perceiving and evaluating body images. For example, there are significant brain responses when you merely show women simple line drawings of underweight, normal weight and overweight female bodies.[16] But when women are encouraged to compare themselves with other women's body shapes things go downhill emotionally and neurologically. A multinational team of scientists published a study in *NeuroImage,* the title of which says it all: 'I'm not as slim as that girl: Neural bases of body shape self-comparison to media images.' They showed images of slim, idealised bodies and interior designs to healthy females between sixteen and thirty-five years old and encouraged them to compare their own body shape and home with those in the images. Unlike the neutral effects of looking at images of interior designs, images of slim women immediately activated the brain's body-shape processing networks to assess the body size and shape of the woman in the photo. However, a second related 'emotional' brain network then kicks in, which deals with the comparison between your body and the slender model/actress/dancer/singer/general celeb in the photo and, most importantly, your *emotional* reaction to the outcome of that comparison, which is unlikely to end happily. And for these women it certainly didn't, as the slender images produced 'dynamic activations of the fear network', along with other brain networks involving less than comforting emotions.

So even in healthy women, the team concluded, 'Brain networks associated with anxiety induced by self-comparison to slim images may be involved in the genesis of body dissatisfaction and hence with vulnerability to eating disorders.'[17]

And when the images get personal, female brains begin to hot up, reacting somewhat violently to the idea that a woman may be slightly heavier than she'd like. By showing men and women distorted images of their own bodies (fat, real and thin versions), an interesting study in *Biological Psychiatry* found that, 'Women tend to perceive distorted images of their own bodies by complex cognitive processing of emotion, whereas men tend to perceive distorted images of their own bodies by object visual processing and spatial visual processing.'[18] And this theme of women's brains having a far more emotional reaction to body images is found in other studies. Researchers at Hiroshima University presented healthy women and those with eating disorders with morphed images of themselves and that of another woman. The prefrontal cortex and the amygdala (areas of the brain implicated in processing emotional reactions such as fear, threat, anxiety and emotional responses to pain) were 'significantly activated [in] healthy women in response to their own fat-image'.[19]

Increased activation of the brain's medial prefrontal cortex (mPFC) can suggest extreme unhappiness and, in some cases, self-loathing. In one study healthy women with a high degree of body confidence looked at images of avatar-like models in skimpy bikinis: some overweight, some very thin. With each image, the women were told to imagine that someone else was saying the model looked like her. When presented with over-weight images, the mPFC showed increased activation in *all* of the women. Merely imagining that they might be overweight seemed to lead women to question their sense of self, even though they claimed afterward that the test was boring or meaningless. Men showed no significant mPFC activation while processing equivalent male images. The researchers concluded that there are 'sub-clinical' issues with body image among healthy women and a much finer line between women with and without eating disorders than previously thought. The lead researcher commented, 'This is kind of validating the suspicion that most women are teetering on the edge of an eating disorder.'[20]

Even the printed word elicits similar neurological reactions in women. The Japanese study 'Gender differences in brain activity generated by unpleasant word stimuli concerning body image' found that in women, words such as 'obesity', 'corpulence' or 'heavy' were accompanied by increased activation in the amygdala, while the areas associated with decision-making and rational thought became inactive. In men the response was the reverse. The authors believe that the mPFC is responsible for the gender differences in the processing of words concerning

body image, and possibly also for gender differences in susceptibility to eating disorders.[21] On the other side of the world,
German psychologists put electrodes on women and looked for
their physiological 'startle responses' when they read neutral
words and 'body words' (e.g. hips, thighs, arms, legs, roll of
flab, etc.). Women with higher levels of body dissatisfaction had
greater startle responses when they saw body-related words.[22]

If 'healthy' women are so easily affected by idealised images
and body-related words, think of how much more vulnerable
girls and women may be distressed by the normal daily
onslaught of media images and messages.

As visual media of thin female physiques reaches further
across the globe, the neurological reactions cited above may be
occurring among growing sections of the world's population,
and at younger ages, helping body discontent to become even
more normative.

The upshot of this neurology is that the body images we
expose ourselves to can have concrete mechanical effects on the
way our brains function and can cause medical problems. This
new evidence should galvanise women's efforts to protect themselves and their children from the intensity of the unhealthy
idealised images we've tolerated for too long. What may seem
an ephemeral bit of light aesthetic fluff can be insidiously
harmful and, in vulnerable people, even fatal.

High dose of images

The rise in the number of idealised images we're exposed to
daily compared with our grandparents is utterly unimaginable.
And it isn't just the content – it's also the sheer number of
images that is doing our heads in.

In addition to the large quantity of figure-obsessed celeb
magazines and newspapers containing tremendous pictorial

content, in a relatively short space of time we've gone from four television stations to hundreds, plus the facility to record programmes or watch DVDs. And then, of course, there are all the images – still and moving – on the Internet. At the moment the average adult watches an average of four hours and twenty minutes of television a day – that's thirty hours a week. At this rate, by the time they're seventy-five the average Briton will have spent more than twelve years' worth of twenty-four-hour days just watching television. And they won't be seeing many size 12s there. Added to this, by the time the average child today is seven, they've already spent a full year's worth of twenty-four-hour days watching recreational screen media.

You couldn't make it up: the American Academy of Pediatrics has recently published a report on 'The Impact of Social Media on Children, Adolescents and Families', which contains a section entitled 'Facebook Depression' (defined as 'depression that develops when preteens and teens spend a great deal of time on social media sites, such as Facebook, and then begin to exhibit classic symptoms of depression').[23] The intensity of social comparisons is one of the reasons they believe this link exists. When discussing how media affects us, doctors now refer to a 'dose–response relationship' between the numbers of hours spent viewing and the psychological effects this may have on us. In terms of the numbers of idealised body images we're consuming per hour and per day – we've overdosed.[24]

Keeping up

In the greater scheme of things, such intensive exposure to idealised slender images can be described as a new evolutionary pressure potentially tampering with our future development. High exposure to these images alters women's perception of their own sexual attractiveness and mating viability through an ongoing yet subconscious social comparison process referred to as the 'contrast effect'.[25]

In terms of evaluating our own attractiveness, we appear more attractive when contrasted with a person less attractive than us and less attractive when contrasted with someone more attractive than us. Until recently, these self-evaluations of body attractiveness involved comparisons with a relatively small number of other women in the local mating pool, e.g. your cave, village, neighbourhood, school, workplace ... Pizza Hut.

However, today's culture is unique: the points of comparison provided by visual media which women now use in their self-evaluations are not only plentiful and all-pervading, but are demographically atypical, with no relevance to the area in which they live, the circles they move in or even the country in which they are resident. Tens of thousands of idealised, airbrushed images are shipped in, arriving ready for comparison in the brain, from New York, Sydney, Paris, Milan, Tokyo and, of course, Hollywood, showing women who are certainly *not* part of the local 'mating pool'. Worse yet, these images are often of famous women.

We are biologically pre-programmed to be fascinated by status and celebrity. Even rhesus monkeys share this impulse, preferring to watch monkeys of status on television as opposed to common apes or rhesus riff-raff. However, the degree to which we are exposed to famous people has increased dramatically, and the great and the good of today are more physically unrepresentative and slimmer than ever before. And while we prefer to believe that celebrities don't influence us, research paints an entirely different picture.

Fame on the brain

Our brains appear to assign a small set of brain cells to remember specific celebrities that are relevant to us. A group of scientists from UCLA, Caltech and University of Leicester have been using microelectrodes to study how individual brain cells in our hippocampus, known to be involved in memory, respond to images of celebrities when displayed on a laptop. For example, in a person who happened to be a football fan, they found a brain cell that responded to Argentine player Diego Armando Maradona; with a patient obsessed with the *Rocky* films, they tried different characters from the series until they found a brain cell that fired when they showed an image of Mr. T (from *Rocky III*). They showed many photos of Maradona (in different environments, with different background colours, in different postures, with different clothing, etc.) to see if the brain cell responded equally to all the photos, in other words, to the *concept* of Maradona, or only to that particular photograph. And they found that it indeed responded to the concept.

The first and by far the most famous of these brain cells was one that responded to seven completely different images of the actress Jennifer Aniston and to no other images. So the cell fired when the person was shown different photos of Aniston, but not when shown celebrities like Julia Roberts, Oprah Winfrey or Pamela Anderson, places like the Golden Gate Bridge or the Eiffel Tower or different animals.[26] Stranger than science fiction.

A study at the University of Houston wanted to zero in on the role of fame in influencing body dissatisfaction – does a famous skinny celeb make you feel worse about your body than an unfamiliar skinny model? Young women saw familiar thin celebrities or familiar moderately overweight celebrities, as well as unfamiliar images of thin or moderately overweight non-celebrity models. Seeing well-known slim celebrities clearly had a negative effect on the young women's body satisfaction 'significantly larger than any other … the greatest effect'. However, images of overweight celebrities did not cause body dissatisfaction. The researchers suspect this may be because the participants were seeing an example of another woman who does not fit the thin ideal, yet was able to find 'success'. They suggest that this could reduce anxiety about one's own body.

So according to the study, when the contrast effect meets fame, the ratings for your body satisfaction may drop: 'celebrities may have more power to influence how a woman feels about her body than just an unknown model … the current trend in Hollywood to cast almost exclusively underweight actresses may be seriously contributing to the feelings of anxiety that many women feel today.'

By the way, the author complained, 'In fact, it was difficult to find many images of celebrities who were not extremely skinny for this study.'[27]

In short, from an increasingly earlier age, women today are exposed to evolutionarily novel points of comparison that deceive their finely honed mental and neurological processes whose function developed over 200,000 years, to evaluate other women in a small-scale local mating pool. The result is the widespread body-image distortion and dissatisfaction reported above. Hollywood may indeed be making history, but not in the way we expected. Life today for many women has evolved to become a case of 'keeping up with the Boneses'.

Perhaps instead of trying to lose weight, it's time to go on a media diet.

Four

What Men Want

... he liked plumpness in a woman, the flesh that takes in the sharp edges and splinters of a man's fate.

Nadine Gordimer, 2002

On the night they become pregnant, nearly 60 per cent of women in the US and half of Australian women are obese or overweight.[1]

Every minute of the day a large proportion of fat women are sexually attractive to men to the point of getting pregnant. This often repeats itself, and the overweight woman is likely to be fatter each time her partner is turned on enough to impregnate her one more time.

Governments are so concerned with men's continuing desire for these fat, fertile women that they are taking pre-emptive measures. Britain's National Institute for Health and Care Excellence states that 'as the number of obese mothers soars', new advice on weight management is being issued before they get pregnant.[2]

While all of this sex and reproduction is going on, women are led to believe that body fat is ugly and sexually unattractive. So clearly, either someone is lying or men must simply be kind, submitting to charitable sexual encounters with these unattractive creatures out of genuine pity and compassion.

I don't think so.

When we try to establish a universal healthy yardstick on female body size and shape, evaluating the types of female body men prefer is a valid and highly important perspective. Knowing what men want can actually serve as an antidote to the prevailing assumptions that feed body dissatisfaction. Therefore, whether you consider it politically incorrect or not, it is a real part of life and history and will not be going away any time soon.

The Totem Pole of Truth

You may not be able to trust a man, but you can trust a part of him that rarely lies. Researchers have been busy carrying out 'penis response profiling' through 'phallometric assessment' of men's 'erotic preferences' or, as other scientists put it, 'genital arousal to stimuli depicting their preferred sex partners'. In other words, they monitor the blood flow and swelling in a man's penis as he views photos and videos of people, naked or otherwise, as a barometer of the extent to which he gets turned on by what he sees.

And according to his wired-up sexual barometer, it seems that what he says he fancies is what he honestly does fancy: 'the relationship between genital responses and reported feelings of sexual arousal in men is positive and large'. Or, put simply, the men's minds and genitals were in agreement over what turned them on.[3] And they were offered quite a menu to consider. Straight men swelled while looking at heterosexual or lesbian sex and while watching naked women masturbate or exercise. They were unmoved when the screen displayed only men. Gay men were aroused in the opposite way – naked, sweaty women weren't exactly their idea of an aphrodisiacal day out. And men of all orientations showed no sexual arousal when watching film of 'bonobo chimpanzee copulation'.[4]

Other studies have added a soundtrack to accompany naked pictures of pre-pubescent girls, pubescent girls, adult women, pre-pubescent boys, pubescent boys and adult men, and clearly found that it was the images of fully sexually mature women that elicited the highest sexual response in heterosexual men, while pre-pubescent and even pubescent girls certainly did not.[5] The main difference that men perceive between a pre-pubescent/pubescent girl versus a sexually viable adult woman is the accumulation of body fat on her hips, thighs and bottom as she reaches full adulthood. These are the secondary sexual characteristics that develop with puberty, which widens the pelvis and increases the amount of body fat in hips, thighs, buttocks and breasts. Interestingly, new studies measuring men's eye movements in response to 'sexually relevant stimuli' support the findings regarding their phallic movements.[6]

As you'll see below, scientists may continue to debate which body parts and pattern of female fat distribution men prefer, but one thing is clear: contrary to cultural and media messages, the vast majority of men most certainly do not find female body fat at all aversive.

Our culture has skewed women's perceptions of what men actually like. For example, when asked to predict how men will rate the attractiveness of women with different body shapes, women choose slimmer figures than men do, figures more like fashion models. The shapes that men *actually* choose are closer to those of the women making the incorrect predictions. Women are often more like men's ideals than they realise, and so by losing weight they may not make themselves any more attractive to them.

Terms and Conditions

While discussing sexual attraction in this way can be seen as merely an excuse to be male, juvenile and facetious, it's actually a necessary part of a reality check on body dissatisfaction. And if it sounds cold, technical and presumptuous to objectify your body by discussing hip and thigh fat and the ratios between your 'inflection points' (key dips and curves on your waist, hips and bust), it's certainly not meant to. Rather, it's meant to demystify and counter the perverse and pervasive messages about female body shape that continue to dominate our culture.

I am most certainly not replacing one prescriptive view of the ideal female form with another. Far from it. This chapter is trying to make clear that men do not find women's body fat ugly, which is certainly not the same as telling women how they should look. Rather, it's saying almost all women have body fat on their hips, thighs and bottoms and, despite media messages to the contrary, men certainly don't find this unattractive. It's saying, you look this way already and often it's fine.

For those who complain that not all men like hip and thigh fat and, that I do not acknowledge a preference in some men for women with a very thin figure with minimal hip, thigh and bottom fat, I do, of course, recognise that this is so. However, I'm trying to counteract the prevailing highly damaging generalisation that female body fat is unattractive and disliked by men. And I am correct in generalising about what the vast majority of men prefer, without discounting or criticising the views of a minority of others.

Blind Man's Buff

The role of visual media has dominated discussions about the female waist and hip body-fat distribution and shape that women think is sexually attractive. And it is also assumed that visual media determine men's sexual preferences in women's body shape: those women who conform to 'social standards of beauty'.

However, evolutionary psychologists suspect that such a fundamental process is not created by visual media, but that it has a far more profound basis, infinitely more established than TV or magazines. And so to test the true nature of men's 'mate preferences' a clever study published in *Evolution and Human Behavior* asked men who had never seen a woman or even a TV or a magazine in their life because they were born blind, to rate the attractiveness of female body shapes on a scale of one to ten, based upon touch and feel alone.

The result of the 'body Braille' touchy-feely study found that blind men certainly do not find hip fat unsexy and actually prefer a more pear-shape fat distribution 'in the complete absence of visual input and, hence, that such input is not necessary for the preference to develop'. By the way, when the researchers asked fully sighted men who were blindfolded, they got a similar result and when they allowed fully sighted men to look and touch too, the preference for pear-shape hip fat was even stronger. 'Our blind participants' WHR [waist-to-hip ratio] preferences were *certainly* not directly shaped by visual media exposure, but they none the less expressed a clear preference for low WHR.'

The scientists think that media images reinforce and fine-tune men's pre-existing preferences.[7] Men may have an evolved neurobiological predisposition to find sexually attractive the very hip, thigh and butt fat that designers, fashion editors and casting directors deplore and the diet industry charges money to get rid of. And remember how honest men are when it comes to what they fancy. Men have known exactly what they want for millennia. But why do they swell at the sight of a swollen-looking physique?

Sexual Dimorphism

Sexual dimorphism – the systematic difference in body shape between males and females – is *central* to sexual attraction and selecting your mate. In females, this means having more subcutaneous fat and fat deposits, mainly around the buttocks, thighs and hips compared to a man or a pubescent girl. That hated pear shape again.

Part of the function of sexual dimorphism is that at a most basic level it works as a cue for sex identification and denotes otherness, i.e. that you are the *opposite* sex to a man. Studies of 'sex identification via waist-to-hip ratio' find that when you remove other visual clues to a person's sex, both men and women look at waist-to-hip fat distribution to determine if someone is male or female. As hips become bigger compared to waists, people are more and more likely to identify that figure as being female.[8]

Interestingly, men with lower, more feminine waist-to-hip ratios (WHRs) feel less comfortable and self-report lower body satisfaction and self-efficacy (one's own ability to complete tasks and reach goals) than men with higher, more masculine WHRs.[9]

But beyond indicating to a man that you are a woman, your hip, thigh and buttock fat serves as a resumé when he is subconsciously evaluating the prospect of a relationship with you.

Generally, women's waist-to-hip ratio is very strongly related to male perception of female attractiveness across all cultures and throughout history. It is a key health and fertility indicator and core feature of feminine beauty.[10]

But how exactly can the fat on your hips, thighs and buttocks speak to men and what does it tell them? Researchers at the Department of Epidemiology, University of Pittsburgh may have found one intriguing answer. They noted that in a cross-cultural study of fifty-eight societies, 'fatter legs and hips in females were valued in 90 per cent [of societies]'. They also noted that gluteo-femoral fat (the fat on your hips, thighs and buttocks) contains long-chain polyunsaturated fatty acids, critical for the development of a foetus's brain. In their study 'Waist-hip ratio and cognitive ability: is gluteofemoral fat a privileged store of neurodevelopmental resources?' the answer seems to be yes – a foetus may benefit intellectually from a mother's hip fat. These findings suggest that 'gluteofemoral fat reflects the availability of neurodevelopmental resources and thus offer a new explanation for men's preference for low WHR'.[11]

Another study of 'Body Configuration in Women' found that women with more gluteofemoral fat (low WHR) 'excel at identifying emotional states of other people and show a cognitive style that favors empathizing'. So more feminine pear-shaped body types (a low WHR) are linked with a more female 'brain type', possessing qualities such as the ability to read another person's mental state and to empathise with them because both qualities may depend upon the effects of female oestrogens at puberty. The researchers think this brain benefit is down to greater gluteofemoral fat stores which are high in the essential fatty acids needed to support brain development and brain cell functioning.

And for the particularly curvy woman who, the researchers say, is 'more likely to be targeted for dishonest courtship' there's an added benefit to her enhanced mind-reading talents.

She 'may be better at identifying disingenuous claims of commitment', thereby protecting herself from a scenario of bump and dump.[12]

So it may be that a man has a longer-term selfish stake in his woman's fat distribution: both he and his child will be better cared for (greater empathy and ability to identify emotional states) and the child may also end up with intellectual advantages. Yet all the while, the media promotes the opposite message: that being lean and mean, fit and toned is more likely to offer benefits for man and baby.

Lesbian and Bisexual Women

It's interesting to add another point of comparison and body-shape judgment: that of lesbian and bisexual women. Straight men and lesbians are strange bedfellows when it comes to what female body shapes they like. Both also seem to be more 'tolerant' toward straight women's weight and shape than straight women are themselves.

For instance, a recent review of the evidence, 'Body image in homosexual persons', found that 'homosexual women are ... more satisfied with their bodies while being more tolerant to obesity ... For lesbian women the ideal body image is more massive than for heterosexual women.'[13]

Two studies at the University of Pennsylvania, 'Lesbian and bisexual women's judgments of the attractiveness of different body types', found that 'in both studies, a heavy figure with a low waist-to-hip ratio was most preferred'.[14] And a study in England ticked all four boxes in their investigation into 'Physical Attractiveness Preferences of Feminist and Nonfeminist Heterosexual Women and Lesbians'. Political orientation didn't reveal much: 'Self-identification as a feminist did not appear to be associated with a preference for larger BMIs. However, they did report 'lesbians preferring images of women with significantly higher BMIs than heterosexual women'.[15]

Part of the reason that lesbian and bisexual women appear to be more easygoing than heterosexual women about their bodies has been described in the *Psychology of Women Quarterly* in terms of greater 'empathy toward body and appearance concerns as well as diversity within same-sex attractions'. The authors believe the evidence may indicate that same-sex relationships can encourage women to feel happier with their bodies.[16]

Breasts vs Buttocks: the Body Wars

Arguments continue over precisely what aspects of the female form are more important in attracting men. Issues such as breast vs buttocks, breast vs waist, hips vs waist, total fat vs distribution of fat and, of course, those mathematical ratios – waist-to-hip ratio (WHR) vs waist-to-buttocks ratio (WTB) – are hotly debated by academics.

In their study 'Perception of female buttocks and breast size in profile' British researchers reported that when exposing men to three varying levels of breast size and three levels of buttock size, 'results showed significant main effects of breast size ... but not of buttock size'.[17]

However, I've discovered that a certain Professor Sigman (no relation), Director of the Integrative Neuroscience Laboratory at the University of Buenos Aires, has taken issue with the buxom British findings. And after reading the title of his fully funded research paper, 'Eye Fixations Indicate Men's Preference for Female Breasts or Buttocks' published in the *Archives of Sexual Behavior*, I realise that I'm the Dr Sigman who drew the short research straw. My observant namesake spotted a gap in the literature – 'There is little empirical research that has examined individual differences in male preferences (e.g. favoring breasts over buttocks)' – and he immediately filled it with 'erotic pictures' of women wearing very, very little. His team got straight to work, discovering that 'at higher levels of preference, men preferring buttocks report a more marked preference', exhibiting a clear 'buttocks preference intensity' (PI) score of '>0.8 and, in sharp contrast, only 1 participant had a breast preference with a PI>0.8'.[18]

But a butt is not a butt unless it's viewed at the correct angle, according to researchers at Harvard. When measuring men's sexual preferences in female body shape, experimental techniques using 'frontal pictures' exclude the buttocks. To remedy the situation, the experimenters gave men more choice by adding sideways profile pictures of women, including some with 'more protruding buttocks ... with the ratio of the waist to buttocks varying'. Everyone was happy as the experiment concluded that men from the Hadza hunter–gatherers in northern Tanzania preferred 'more protruding buttocks' than American men.[19]

So in considering what men want, we can be preoccupied with body parts and ratios, but again it's clear that the appeal of female body fat is not merely at the whim of media fashion; there is a longstanding universal appreciation of it by men across time and space for good evolutionary reasons.

Everybody Needs a Bosom for a Pillow

Arguing about body parts and fat ratios just got even more complicated because men's preferences for female body shape can vary slightly according to the local geography of the society they live in or their economic circumstances.

In this age of plenty we have to be reminded of the fact that a primary function of body-fat tissue is the storage of calories – like a fuel tank. At a primitive level, this can mean that body fat is a reliable predictor of food availability. And so for men, even today, seeing female body fat may still signal a sense of 'resource security'. Heavier female body sizes are preferred where or when resources are unpredictable or unavailable. Hungry men prefer significantly heavier women than satiated men – not because they want them in the stew pot.

When socioeconomic or individual conditions are threatening or uncertain, individuals will prefer others with more mature physical characteristics, including a heavier body size. For example, American actresses with more mature facial and bodily features are more popular during periods of socioeconomic hardship because physical maturity is associated with the ability to handle threatening situations; more mature physical features may communicate attributes such as strength, control and independence during periods when such qualities should be most desired.

Getting back to the here and now, British research on 'The Impact of Psychological Stress on Men's Judgements of Female Body Size' clearly found that 'men experiencing stress not only perceive a heavier female body size as maximally attractive, but also more positively perceive ... heavier female bodies as more attractive and idealised a wider range of female figures'.[20] The researchers then zeroed in on bosoms with an international follow-up study, 'Resource Security Impacts Men's Female Breast Size Preferences'. It has been suggested that human female breast size may act as a signal of fat reserves which, in turn, indicates access to resources.

The researchers asked 1266 men from three areas in Malaysia of varying relative socioeconomic status (high to low) to rate various breast sizes for physical attractiveness. 'Results showed that men from the low socioeconomic context rated larger breasts as more attractive than did men from the medium socioeconomic context, who in turn perceived larger breasts as more attractive than men from a high socioeconomic context.' Back in Britain the scientists compared the breast-size preferences of sixty-six hungry men versus fifty-eight who were satiated. The results showed that the hungry men rated larger breasts as significantly more attractive. 'Taken together, these studies provide evidence that resource security impacts upon men's attractiveness ratings based on women's breast size.'[21]

A strange insight into the body shapes that men like came in a private study which claimed to have mapped out a billion Internet searches by measuring web traffic of more than 100 million people around the world. The researchers concluded that a woman's body size appears to be a powerful trigger for male arousal. Adjectives that describe body size (e.g. 'chubby' or 'thin') are the third most common category of adjectives found in the Internet searches they analysed. It turned out that most of these searches were not looking for svelte model shapes at all. In fact, for every search for a 'skinny' girl, there were, apparently, almost three for a 'fat' girl. They identified more than 504 adult sites explicitly dedicated to heavy ladies, and only 182 to thin ones. They delicately explain that the women on the bigger-woman websites sites 'have very large and round breasts, large and curvy hips, and large and round butts. Indeed, the overall impression is one of supersize visual cues of femininity.'[22]

Aural Sex

Stepping back from the minutiae of the breast/buttocks wars, other researchers believe that a man does not view a woman's body as just a modular structure comprised of a collection of hips, thighs, buttock, bosoms and inflection points, but instead forms a general impression whereby the whole is greater than the sum of its parts. This is an example of the *gestalt effect*: our bias to look for figures and whole forms, instead of just a collection of simple lines and curves. In their 'penile response' study, 'Sexual Attraction to Others ... alloerotic responding in men', Canadian researchers came to the conclusion that 'men respond to a potential sexual object as a gestalt, which they evaluate in terms of global similarity to other potential sexual objects'.[23] So you may be a sex object, but he is taking into consideration the whole person.

But irrespective of the holistic 'gestalt' impression a man has of your body, there are many other important aspects to your being that he is attracted to. Like your body, the sound of your voice also has a shape – a sonic silhouette that provides men with information. And, like body shape, it is also a secondary sexual characteristic.[24] Men tend to agree strongly about *which* voices are attractive. But they have trouble pinpointing exactly what it is that attracts them.

How attractive men find women's voices has been found to vary across the menstrual cycle. For example, female voices are perceived by some men as more attractive closer to ovulation,[25] when women are most fertile, and less so premenstrually, while one study concluded that 'voices recorded at menstruation were identified as being the most unattractive'.[26]

Voice characteristics such as the width of your 'formant dispersion', 'roundness' of your 'glottal waveforms', and, of course, your fundamental frequency – coupled with your other speech characteristics – create an immediate sonic image. And that's not even taking into consideration your accent, diction and *what* you are saying, for, as one linguist put it, 'Language puts minds on display'.

If you don't believe me, consider this: most Western countries today have advertisements for expensive phone lines that men can ring to hear a 'sexy woman/hot babe' talk to them; it's known as 'phone sex'. According to the experts, 'It doesn't matter if you are old or young, black or white, or heavy or skinny; it is the voice that counts the most.'[27]

The key attractions of a 'phone-sex professional' are her voice and her sexual role-play skills, along with the experienced ability to discern and respond to a customer's needs. A man can ring agency switchboards and the receptionist will try to find a suitable woman – one with the right-shaped voice – to call him back. So male sexual attraction is clearly about more than merely your body shape. Sonic body satisfaction, perhaps?

Nurturing/Caring

When you think of a sexual advisor or dating coach for women, the name Bill Bryson doesn't immediately come to mind, yet after reading how he was initially attracted to, fell in love with and married his wife of thirty-eight years, I'd highly recommend him as one.

When Bryson took up work in a psychiatric hospital in Surrey all those years ago, he noticed a nurse tending to and feeding a dribbling patient. And that was it – her nurturing had him hooked.

Nurses' uniforms are about as different to lap-dancer wear as you can get, yet they are often considered sexy, and are sold in party and adult sex shops. Why? It certainly isn't because of the revealing design.

Men often find nurses – and teachers or carers of young children – very attractive or, as some men put it, 'They have a strong reputation as wife material'. One man I spoke to said, 'There is something about women being nice to old people, children and guys they aren't interested in that makes men feel reassured about their compatibility as relationship partners and potential wives.'

And for those of you with more malevolent intentions, remember too that when Samson let his guard down and got his unexpected crew-cut it was because he was being nurtured by Delilah: 'And she made him sleep upon her knees; and she called for a man, and she caused him to shave off the seven locks of his head; and she began to afflict him, and his strength went from him.'

There seems to be a paucity of research or even a conscious awareness of this subsonic bass note of attraction. But I imagine the appeal of caring and nurturing has a relatively straightforward explanation. Asking around to hear Representative Man's thoughts I was told:

All men come from women, and that nurturing that we received as a baby imprints on us, and try as we like, we can't get away from that.

Mr Average

A man knows that the pressure is on for him to stay large and in charge in the world, and it's a real anxiety-inducer for him to consider what might happen to his relationship if he hits some bumps in the road. If he's with a nurturing woman, he can trust that if and when he does slip, he'll get compassionate encouragement instead of negative reinforcement.

Mr Standard

She'll be nurturing to the kids. Maybe it's subconsciously because we want to further our family tree. It could also remind us of our moms, and we know that she raised us well, so this woman would raise your kids well. Again, back to furthering the family tree.

Mr Guy Regular

What Men Want

All men want to be looked after. Or we just like being babied.

Mr Matt Nappy

Of course, there are masochistic men brought up by unrespon-sive, cold mothers who will take issue with the idea that most men find caring women more appealing. Ignore them unless you're knowingly sadistic or are simply looking to establish a dysfunctional relationship.

In a curious twist of redressing past inequities between men and women, the media has portrayed women as behaving more in the way men have traditionally behaved. Apparently, once women are freed from the social and economic constraints suf-fered before, they naturally behave in a more masculine way. They 'have balls' and 'kick ass'. As women's bodies have become leaner and harder on television and film, so has their accompanying behaviour. It's as if a sense of physical, emotional and behavioural otherness is being played down. For example, it's now less fashionable to portray women as caring and nurtur-ing toward a man. Perhaps media culture considers these images as akin to showing a woman being servile, deferential and weak, or in some way compromising her independence. Or perhaps it's simply uncool to be caring, and nurturing is badly lacking in edginess. Yet it's precisely these caring, nurturing qualities that make the world a bearable place.

After centuries of women being seen as little more than non-voting sex objects and baby factories, society has understandably placed an increasing emphasis on a woman's accomplishments. But this has become confused with and misinterpreted as being the qualities that act as a woman's sexual appeal. The two are not the same. When it comes to romance, it's not your list of credentials that impresses men – it's how they feel about them-selves when they're with you. One male 'dating coach' and author of the indelicately entitled *Why He Disappeared* advises plainly: 'If you think that he's going to be drawn to you for your *accomplishments* – your degree, your job, your home, your impressive hobbies – you're really missing something fundamental to men ... Understand, men *do* value intelligence, but they also want from their girlfriend what they *can't* get from their business associates. Warmth, affection, nurturing, thoughtfulness.'

This isn't scientific and isn't meant to be, but it's what I've observed around the world – without exception.

It is no coincidence that nearly 85 per cent of counsellors and psychotherapists are female and an American Psychological Association report about the lack of male psychologists is entitled 'Men: A growing minority?'[28] Curiously, society isn't up in arms at this glaring sexual inequality in male representation in these professions. This may be because we unconsciously assume that women dominate in these fields because when it comes to the listening profession in particular women may enjoy it more and be better at it. Indeed, a great deal of research has found that women excel in tests measuring interpersonal sensitivity.[29]

In a publication of the American Psychological Association, Professor D. C. Geary concluded that females are more sensitive to non-verbal communication than males. He argued that 'in comparison to men, the greater emotional reactivity of women might then complement a greater sensitivity to the social cues and the nuances of social relationships. In combination, these competencies will provide women with a relative advantage in managing social relationships.'

Many other scientists, such as Shelley Taylor, have identified characteristics that make women good parents and close friends – characteristics such as becoming anxious when hearing about the problems of friends and acquaintances and heightened sensitivity (compared to men) to emotional facial cues. In one study – 'Tend and Befriend' – she and her colleagues pointed out that, under conditions of stress, 'the desire to affiliate with others is substantially more marked among females than among males' and that this is 'one of the most robust gender differences in adult human behavior'.

Researchers using functional magnetic resonance imaging (fMRI) to study brain activation have found that men and women respond differently to positive and negative stimuli. Women's brain activity suggests a stronger involvement of the neural circuit associated with identifying emotional stimuli, and they also direct more attention to the feelings produced by these.[30]

In short, women have a gift that can't be photographed, manufactured, bottled and sold. It's not a coincidence that one of the best-kept secrets in all areas of the media is that simple caring and kindness are an enormous subliminal sexual attractant to men. These are the female qualities that make a man fall in love.

Non-verbal Communication

Irrespective of how fat or skinny your body is, how it moves also has an influence on attraction. Entire books are written on the influence of non-verbal communication ('body language') and how men respond to it. The German scientist Dr Bernhard Fink and his team examined the potential effect of women's gait on how attractive men found them. Their study – 'Women's body movements are a potential cue to ovulation' – observed that a woman moves differently according to how fertile she is within the menstrual month, and that men notice the difference and may find her more attractive as a result. It seemed to be the 'sway' or 'wiggle' of the hips that did things to men.[31]

If men are blind to your body movements, there is evidence that they may pick up on the way you smell. A study published in *Psychological Science* reported that men who sniffed women's 'ovulation-scented shirts displayed higher levels of testosterone than men who sniffed the non-ovulation or control shirts ... but other studies suggest the testosterone effects are large enough to produce changes in behaviour ... so it stands to reason that a man is more likely to be attracted to an ovulating female and to pursue her as a partner.'[32]

And then there's a body of research and, more importantly, evidence from real life that the movement of eyelashes, body posture, the angle and degree of gaze, facial movements and reactions and, of course, smile all add to the complex chemistry of your attraction or lack of it. So in trying to understand sex appeal, focusing on weight and shape is terribly misguided and badly flawed.

Chubby Chasers

If body fat is such a turn-off, why is there a growing business enabling men to meet 'Plus-sized' women? The international organisation Large Passions celebrates female body fat with the home page:

Welcome to Large Passions!

Full Figured? Plus Size? Voluptuous? Husky? Fat? Rubenesque? Thick? Obese? Portly? Stout? Round? Big Boned? Pear Shaped? Apple Shaped? Chubby? Bottom Heavy? Top Heavy? Diet Challenged?

Men from New Zealand to Finland, Japan to the USA can pursue women who do not look as though they are suffering from starvation. And following the company's success in accommodating the 'BBW' (Big Beautiful Woman), Large Passions now welcomes 'SSBBW' (Super-size Big Beautiful Woman).

However, the best name in big romance has to be Chubby Chasers. I hit their website as I was writing this and came across a photo of a pretty woman looking for a man who appreciates the more substantial woman. The advert read:

CHEESECAKE4U
Female, 33, Houston Texas USA
Hi, my name is Rose. I am a very **loving, caring** . . .

And the next ad ran:

MAKEMEBELIEVE24
Female, 24, Hutchinson Kansas USA
I am a **caring, compassionate**, hard-working . . .

The marketing terms they both use – 'loving, caring' and 'caring, compassionate' – are a smart move.

Of course, there are more pragmatic reasons for seeking the larger woman as a good investment, literally. The Chinese *Chutian Metro Daily* reports many men are on the lookout for a chubby wife who, if an old Chinese superstition is to be believed, will bring their husbands good luck. In Chinese fortune-telling tradition, particular features in a woman are believed to bring enduring good luck to her husband. For instance, a woman with a round face and rotund figure is allegedly able to ensure for her husband a great fortune.[33]

Not only is it counterproductive to focus as much as we do on the importance of your body in attracting men, but to do so ignores the other part of the equation: the inherent and differing configuration of preferences that each man has – i.e. that it's not all about you; it's also about him and what he may be predisposed to like. If you believe men want someone 'beautiful', remember beauty is, to a great extent, in the eye of the beholder.

More Bounce to the Ounce

NEWS FLASH: MEN across Britain continue to be puzzled by the debate over the pros and cons of bouncy girls, it emerged last night ...

So said the *Daily Mash*, a British 'satirical website which publishes spoof articles, i.e. it is all made-up and is not intended, *in any way whatsoever*, to be taken as factual'. Yet the following spoof article is, for most men, so very true:

As the first size 16 contestant prepares for the Miss England beauty pageant, women said it was an important breakthrough while men said they could not imagine the circumstances in which this lovely big girl would be deemed unattractive.

Nathan Muir, a completely normal person in every way from Hatfield, stressed: 'What the hell are you talking about? She's a cracker and I can say with cast-iron certainty that if I, or any of my friends, were lucky enough to be on top of her you would need a crane to get us off.'

... Martin Bishop, a remarkably ordinary human from Doncaster, said: 'I'll be honest, I don't listen to women all that much, but from what I can gather the debate is, essentially, about attractiveness, and therefore it is reasonable to assume that I, as a man, am the one who is supposed to be attracted.

'We keep saying it until we are blue in the face – for the *love of god*, please gain some weight because we do not want to have sex with someone who looks like a 12-year-old boy.'[34]

Who's to Blame?

If there is such a gulf between the thigh-gap values today's women are haunted by and what most men, lesbian and bisexual women find attractive, it begs the questions how and why – and who's responsible? The how and why will be addressed in Part Two of this book, but it is important at this point to identify some of the movers and shakers in the body-dissatisfaction industry who have helped create this damaging misunderstanding. Girls and women deserve a spotlight to be shone into the darker corners of the manufacturers and purveyors of this thigh-gap pursuit. But men too deserve such an enquiry, as they continue to be unfairly blamed for female body dissatisfaction.

It is true that men's interest in enhanced silicone 'gazongas' may help perpetuate the breast-enlargement industry, but 'body fascism', its attendant self-loathing and hip-and-thigh phobia and the general dieting craze are *not* to be laid at the doorstep of man. Instead, they should be attributed to an unholy alliance of fashion designers and picture editors and, as is the case with every area of lifestyle disease, a confederation of economic interests with shareholders.

Some see the error of their ways, confess and seek redemption. Kirstie Clements, a former editor of *Vogue* Australia, reveals 'the ugly truth behind the glamour'. 'It is too simplistic to blame misogynistic men,' she says. ' ... There are many female fashion editors who perpetuate the stereotype, women who often have a major eating disorder of their own.'

But Clements was not unafflicted by the slender bent, couching her preferences for models in the comfy vernacular of 'healthy' and 'toned'. Despite the fact that the average Australian dress size is 16, Clements, like all fashionistas, has her size calibration set on the very, very low side: 'As a *Vogue* editor, I was of the opinion that we didn't necessarily need to feature size 14-plus [UK size 12] models in every issue ... I see no problem with presenting a healthy, toned Australian size 10 [UK size 8–10].'

In recounting a lunch conversation with a top New York agent, Clements gave a rare insight into the behind-the-scenes body barbarity:

> '"It's getting very serious," she said. She lowered her tone and glanced around to see if anyone at the nearby tables could hear. "The top casting directors are demanding that they be thinner and thinner. I've got four girls in hospital. And a couple of the others have resorted to eating tissues. Apparently, they swell up and fill your stomach."'

The Devil really does wear Prada.

Male views of female fat are entirely different from females'. And far kinder too. Men may indeed be bastards or, as one writer laments, 'Men are selfish pigs. And there aren't enough of them to go around.' But it's a myth that men are largely responsible for female body dissatisfaction – women continue to do a superb job of lowering one another's body confidence without any help from men. And it has to stop.

While women are trying to shed the pounds, most men simply want more bounce to the ounce.

Five

Baby Dissatisfaction

Most of the world's women are or will be mothers. This is true even in Western industrialised countries with readily available birth control and legalised abortion. And until recently this was certainly not considered a visual tragedy.

A Plumper Past

Some of the earliest artists who created figurative prehistoric art from the Upper Palaeolithic period (25,000 BC) in distant parts of the world did not seem to find female fertility or the features of motherhood in the slightest bit unattractive. *The Venus of Willendorf* statuette lets it all hang out. Her large breasts, abdomen and broad waistline in general, along with the detail put into the vulva, have led many academics to interpret the figure as a fertility symbol – or a symbol of the hope for survival, and for the attainment of a well-nourished (and thus reproductively successful) maturity, during the harshest period of the major glaciation in Europe. Meanwhile, her somewhat more slight/svelte older sister, *The Venus of Laussel* bas-relief, has her hand on her extremely ample abdomen (or womb), with large breasts and vulva, all comfortably protected by her well-proportioned hips and thighs.

Giving life and nurturing an infant were traditionally endowed with sanctity. Pregnancy and motherhood should mark a period of détente between a woman and her body image. Yet this truce is being increasingly broken.

The title of a modern book *Does This Pregnancy Make Me Look Fat?* encapsulates the zeitgeist, while the description cuts to the chase: 'People might tell you you're glowing, but you just feel like you're growing.' And when baby finally arrives another writer describes 'the unloved post-bump body, the untidy aftermath of the show'.[1]

While body dissatisfaction may be a 'normative discontent' for all, it is now increasing in pregnant women, particularly those who are of a normal weight.[2] And even women with no prior body-image problems fall prey to body dissatisfaction once they have given birth.

An Australian study of women during late pregnancy and early motherhood found many describing some of the unique aspects of their pregnancy which helped them cope positively with their changing bodies. For example, they told of a 'new sense of meaning in life', placing the wellbeing of their developing baby above the way their bodies looked. They spoke of the joy of maternal experiences such as feeling the baby kick. However, 'these events no longer protected against body dissatisfaction post-birth'.[3]

Meanwhile, although research on postnatal body satisfaction and relationship intimacy has focused almost exclusively on mothers, it's now thought that fathers too are affected by both their own as well as their partner's body dissatisfaction during their child's infancy. Nine months after the birth of their first child, both a mother's and father's levels of 'intimacy satisfaction' are related to their own and their partner's level of body satisfaction.[4] For the majority of couples, the transition from more money, time, sleep and sex to parenthood often introduces new strains to their relationships. Body dissatisfaction may be one unrecognised factor in this. In fact, body dissatisfaction can become an excellent form of postnatal birth control.

Ugly Mommy – Baby Blues

At least two studies indicate that a mother's body dissatisfaction reaches its peak at six months after she gives birth. Women become more likely to report that they feel ashamed of their body. Unsurprisingly, several studies show that women want to return to a 'normal' weight after they give birth. Researchers from the University of Minnesota are expressing concern that this cultural 'thinness mindset could unfortunately have negative repercussions on a mother's mental health'.[5]

But the fallout can affect the baby too as many research studies suggest that women who are preoccupied or less satisfied with their body shape are less likely to breastfeed, and more likely to suffer depressive symptoms or psychological distress. This may contribute to a vicious cycle in which depression provokes body dissatisfaction through diminished self-esteem or overeating, and body dissatisfaction itself lowers self-esteem and contributes to depression. The cycle may heighten a mother's risk of developing eating disorders.[6]

Depression can lead mothers to be non-responsive, inconsistent or to reject their infant, placing the mother–baby attachment at risk. Our approach to close relationships or our *attachment style* is believed to be shaped by our early interactions with our primary carers, in particular our biological mother. Early patterns of a baby's attachment have been shown to be an important influence on their adult social behaviour. So what begins as an apparent aesthetic concern accompanying a pregnancy in 2014 may have repercussions decades later.

Depression

How satisfied – or not – you are with your body shape is now thought to be an important factor in determining whether you develop depressive symptoms during pregnancy. And so drug companies will be sad to hear that some scientists now suggest that 'promoting healthy body image may be a non-pharmacological strategy that offers protective effects against depressive symptoms during pregnancy'.[7]

There is further evidence to suggest that body dissatisfaction becomes heightened after birth as a result of both internal and external pressure on a woman to regain her pre-pregnancy body weight and shape.[8] And so given the strong link between body dissatisfaction and depression during pregnancy, and the high incidence of postnatal depression,[9] body dissatisfaction is increasingly being considered as an important factor in a mother's antenatal care.[10]

A Bigger Pregnancy

Irrespective of body image and satisfaction and the dress sizes pregnant women cannot fit into, excessive body fat is, above all, a straightforward health issue for them and the children they bear. Approximately 60 per cent of adult women in countries such as Britain, Australia and the United States are already overweight or obese and, when they become pregnant, the majority gain excessive weight. This high weight gain is the strongest predictor of whether a mother will go on to be overweight or obese after her pregnancy. Furthermore, gaining excessive weight while you're pregnant increases the risk of your child becoming obese long after you give birth, from their childhood all the way into their adult years, even when you take into consideration other contributory fattening factors.[11]

What's more, body dissatisfaction can exacerbate the problem: there is new research from different parts of the world, including Australia and Iran, suggesting that body dissatisfaction before pregnancy and in early to mid-pregnancy is linked to excessive weight gain during pregnancy.[12] Iranian women, for example, who before pregnancy were more dissatisfied with their body size and wanted to be thinner were, by the end of their pregnancy, actually more likely to end up fatter.[13]

And scientists have finally confirmed the obvious – that 'weight-related teasing during mid-pregnancy' is likely to lead to women 'feeling less attractive and feeling fat during late pregnancy'.[14]

A Booby Trap

According to the World Health Organization, 'Breastfeeding is one of the most effective ways to ensure child health and survival ... WHO recommends mothers worldwide to exclusively breastfeed infants for the child's first six months to achieve optimal growth, development and health.'[15]

Unfortunately, however, body dissatisfaction can sully even this most intimate nurturing act. Women halfway through their pregnancies who had greater levels of body dissatisfaction were found to be more worried that breastfeeding would be embarrassing, concerned about the impact it might have on their bodies and sexuality and less comfortable with feeding in public, according to research by the State University of New York.[16]

On the opposite side of the world in Himeji, Japan a study of 'breastfeeding and perceptions of breast shape changes' found that a mother's concern over possible changes in shape of her breasts was linked with her doing less breastfeeding. The majority of mothers perceived some changes in their breast shape, namely 'lost tension', 'changes in size' and 'sagging'. More than half said that breastfeeding also made their breast shape 'drooping'. The public health researchers believe that 'interventions should be developed to improve breastfeeding rates and duration'.[17]

For all the world's women and children, the link between body dissatisfaction during pregnancy and breastfeeding after birth is now considered as a public health matter.[18]

Body Baggage

If pregnant women and mothers today do experience more body dissatisfaction, how can we explain it? Many scientists describe the phenomenon in abstract terms as 'mid-pregnancy perceived sociocultural pressure to be thin'.[19] Others point to 'the cultural "thinness" mindset'.[20] So we have to first put a face – or, more aptly, a body – to concepts such as 'sociocultural pressures' and 'cultural thinness mindset'.

Given that pregnant women and mothers are female, they start off with the same cultural body baggage as described in Chapter 1, 'Size Matters'. But there have been additional changes in how motherhood itself is viewed, portrayed and experienced in ways that affect how they feel about themselves. I would argue that much of the body dissatisfaction experienced by pregnant women and the mothers of young children today is the voice of their reaction to society's ambivalent view of motherhood. Body dissatisfaction has served as a lightning rod for the changes women have recently experienced and the many anxieties they understandably have over motherhood as viewed by our less than supportive culture. To understand what's gone wrong requires a look through the retrospectroscope with a very wide-angle lens.

Celeb mums

The rise in celebrity culture has been accompanied by our exposure to more pregnant and postnatal celebs. At the same time, thanks to digital technology, it is easier to take photos surreptitiously, the resolution of the image is getting better and better, while the portability of the image file – JPEG, TIFF or GIFF – makes the picture instantly transferable, saleable and available. And, of course, Photoshop makes it quick and easy to focus in on cellulite, stretch marks, pockets of mommy flab and other general 'imperfections' 'caused' by that nasty condition, motherhood.

Taking a spin down celebrity alley immediately puts in perspective the points of comparison women and girls are provided with daily. Upon publication of a pregnant or postnatal celeb's photo, the look of pregnancy and early motherhood is then presented with ambivalence by the media, and regularly treated by columnists, journalists and features/photo editors as something that needs to be battled and beaten into submission. Those celebs who shake off motherhood as quickly as possible are to be revered.

Women have more recently been treated to a backhanded compliment, as the media fetishises the great and the good with a bun in their oven. As the Duchess of Cambridge began to swell, lifestyle magazines talked of the cult of the bump ('bumpophilia'). But it is clearly just another domain in which to judge women's bodies.

A female writer on these matters puts it beautifully: 'Like all matters relating to women's bodies, there is an ideal to be lived up to. And the perfect bump is neat and high. It creates depth, but not width; it does not splurge out to the side or come with a side order of swollen limbs and double chin ... The look we aspire to is python who swallowed a bowling ball.'[21] While that python profile may be nice, instead of looking like a model mommy, you may end up as merely a mound of motherhood.

As in all media insinuation, the pregnant look is seen as an extension of self-control and style, while the reality is you cannot order your bump size and shape, nor the general size and shape of your pregnant body and face by ticking the right boxes on the right online shopping page. Genetics, physiology (including hormones, morning sickness, cravings for pig lard sandwiches as opposed to plums) and the size and number of the babies inside you, will choose your bump profile for you.

The body-image bandits

Carla Bruni, wife of the former French president Nicolas Sarkozy, recently described how she was criticised in the press for her appearance immediately following the birth of her daughter, Giulia. 'They say, "She's fat." They get really nasty. Nothing is out of bounds.' However, Bruni also made clear how she felt as a woman: 'It was a very fragile moment in my life. I'm kind of tall, with good-size shoulders, and when I am forty pounds overweight, I don't even look fat – I just look ugly.'[22]

Most postnatal mothers are treated daily to photos and news such as:

Radiant Jennifer Lopez back in shape just five weeks after giving birth to twins ... with little sign left of the massive 50lb she gained during her pregnancy.[23]

Many mothers reading a bit of celeb gossip to pass the time while breastfeeding and perhaps to kill the pain of the mastitis they're not exactly enjoying, may stumble across snippets from *Time* magazine, for example, showing them how the other half don't live: 'Jennifer Lopez was widely quoted as saying she had decided not to breastfeed her twins.'[24]

And if you're pregnant and can rest an iPad on your bump there are celeb-news websites to help you gauge how you measure up:

'Lose that mummy-tummy and look just like the stars!'

The famous food dodgers' menu of the day may look something like:

Actress **Jessica Alba** used an intensive training regime called the 321 Baby Bulge Be Gone plan and is admired and adored for regaining her toned body. Her other secret? She wore a corset for three months.

She 'ballooned' when she was pregnant into the size of a small house, but **Katie Holmes** famously dropped her baby weight in just five months. She hired a trainer to regain her lost body shape and followed a very strict diet.

Model **Heidi Klum** took photographs of herself nude after her pregnancy as the motivation to stick to her diet, even when she was hungry, and says breast-feeding was the reason she lost weight so quickly.

Christina Aguilera lost 18kg in four months after giving birth, sticking to a strict diet regime and an equally strict fitness routine that involved a 90-minute workout every day.

Kim Kardashian was cruelly compared to a whale when she was pregnant, spurring her on to lose 43 pounds and telling the world it was so 'rewarding' and she was loving being 'back to feeling like myself'.

And inevitably, three months after she'd given birth to Britain's future king, close-ups of the Duchess of Cambridge were accompanied by joyous exclamations of 'Look! No mummy tummy!' and 'Kate's gym-slim!'

In the cold, rational light of day we realise all of the above may be candy-floss fantasy. Of course, in general, we don't like to acknowledge that despite our intelligence and belief in independent thought and 'free will', we are not impervious to an ecosystem of celeb images and ridiculous claims. The net effect of this is feeding an unachievable aspiration to regain your pre-pregnancy look, the 'failure' of which is down to your own lack of self-discipline and general abilities as a mother and woman. It's entirely your fault because you're just a slob. Not.

Motherism

If the television in the 1950s and 60s projected the accommodating, apron-clad, biscuit-baking contented housewife with that Colgate ring of confidence, the past twenty years have wiped that smile off her face. The status of the full-time mother has taken a dive. Today, a 'successful' woman, as depicted by the media, is a slender, young *professional* woman – or just a slender young woman. But the image of a woman whose success is defined through stay-at-home motherhood is conspicuous by its absence. Her situation seems to lack the televisual excitement and immediacy necessary for TV broadcast, so it never even makes it to the casting couch. Full-time motherhood has become déclassé. A status which, understandably, does not lend itself to body confidence.

The political womb

Beyond the visual landscape of flat celebrity abdomens there has been a fundamental change in the way motherhood is considered. Despite the fact that most women – conservative-right or liberal-left – are, or will be, mothers, motherhood has become increasingly politicised and portrayed as a problem to be solved, while child wellbeing is viewed through the prism of sexual politics and women's rights. From contraception to abortion to delivery by scheduled Caesarean section, breast milk to daycare to state benefits to the so-called 'work–life balance' – what was a more unconscious intuitive eventuality for most has become a far more considered affair.

This truly is a brave new world for mothers, many of whom are likely to have had a career for a decade or more before starting a family: this is history in the making. For many women, a career means having some degree of power and influence, and that's certainly reversed at 3 a.m. when there's a baby screaming and their left breast has gone dry. In many ways, life goes from 'intellectual' to primitive and instinctual – it seems like a decided step backward, like going from master to work experience. Often, maternity leave serves as nothing more than a last-minute relief allowing little time to adequately accommodate the transition from working woman to mother. (All in the knowledge that they may well lose their place on the career ladder when they try to return to work.)

And parenting itself has grown more political. The pressure builds, as we are more conscious of what we can, should and should not do to bring about the best 'child outcomes' to accentuate the positive and eliminate the negative. In the space of a few decades the way we parent has changed dramatically, so that something we once did naturally and unthinkingly has become the subject of political fashion, guided by experts.

Misery Mumoirs

When women become mothers, they are often portrayed as creatures who gain a baby and lose a brain. They are said to talk predominantly about changing nappies – as if by talking about nappies a mother is rendered incapable of talking about anything else. Moreover, it becomes increasingly difficult to see the reality that this aspect of motherhood is something you surrender to for a limited period of time during which you may well be immersed in nappies. Motherhood is portrayed as a cul-de-sac along the avenue of real life. Once you set off on that road trip there is an incessant ambient pressure to get back to normal life, 'real' life. Yet giving life is surely about as real and raw as life gets.

The recent transition to greater self-expression has allowed many mothers to write about their feelings and the problems of pregnancy and motherhood to a degree and depth unthinkable only a generation or so ago. This is helpful to those who are reassured that they are not the only ones less than entirely happy with their current state. Or as the late commentator Cathy Crimmins shared, 'A period is just the beginning of a lifelong sentence'. The highlight of this lifelong sentence is shared by another happy mum, Sherry Glaser who offers these comforting words to prospective mothers: 'I realise why women die in childbirth – it's preferable.'

Yet for most women motherhood is relatively uneventful,

characterised by its mundaneness. And so the snappy, sharp 'if-it-bleeds-it-reads'-style pieces written by media-mum columnists do not reflect the real lives of most mothers in most countries, the majority of whom derive much of the meaning of their lives ... from being mothers. How awful.

To add insult to injury, many mothers feel less attractive and less interesting. It seems as though they feel that if they were working again, they would regain control over their lives, along with the esteem that has gone missing. And there are ubiquitous role models to help this process along. Given the way appearance and form have taken precedence over deeper content, the image of the modern, slender, well-dressed and groomed professional woman in heels, toting an iPhone 5, while sliding into her new VW Beetle is sleek, up-to-date and aspirational. And as a snapshot of success and empowerment, it is more persuasive and seductive than a tired mother in a smock with baby poo on her right thumb.

If men were to undergo all of the above changes and experience the negative or ambivalent feelings associated with them, they might react with erectile dysfunction or perhaps even a mass killing spree of the type we see on the news. But in women this can be subtly expressed through body dissatisfaction.

A Rebirth of Motherhood

Despite growing evidence that body dissatisfaction is prevalent among pregnant women,[27] and that it is linked with a range of not so very nice effects on women's health[28] (including depression, obesity and excessive pregnancy weight gain for the mother, as well as unhealthy eating behaviours that can negatively impact on the unborn child's future health and development), it has, until recently, been largely ignored by healthcare professionals working with pregnant women. This will hopefully change further as awareness is growing.

Our grandmothers wouldn't have needed the difference between their bodies before having children and after explained to them in sensitive detail. But now doctors are adamant that it is important to educate women about the bodily changes, including weight gain and the realistic expected course of postnatal weight loss and further changes, and to find ways to enhance a mother's body image and self-esteem after she gives birth.[29]

Changing society's and individual women's perceptions of pregnancy and motherhood will take time and pressure, but I believe a change in focus and perspective can be achieved. And a change in perspective (and expectations) may have significant effects on the way women view their bodies in future. An interesting insight into this process was revealed in a study by the Department of Woman and Child Health at the Karolinska Institute, Stockholm where body dissatisfaction in women who became pregnant through IVF was compared with those who became pregnant without it. Interestingly, women previously told they were otherwise infertile, yet who then became pregnant through IVF treatment 'experienced their pregnancies in a less negative way ... IVF women were less negative about their pregnant body ... and they were also less worried about possible "loss of freedom" in their future lives as parents.'[30]

Think about it, from gay people to disabled people, we have revolutionised the way society views a wide variety of groups of human beings. Given that more than half the world's population are female and most have been, are or will be pregnant, there is an overwhelming vested interest in a revolution in our view of pregnancy and motherhood from the top (politically) down. Mothers of young children are usually busy, tired and overstretched and therefore don't have the political voice their number and role deserves. We have to ensure their voice is heard and that our governments are fitted with a hearing aid with the volume turned up loud.

If body dissatisfaction has functioned as a voice expressing unease over the changes women have recently experienced and the many anxieties they understandably have over motherhood as undermined by our culture, it isn't just their feelings and wellbeing today that are at stake. This current devalue system may also set in motion a maternal role-modelling effect in which children learn that pregnancy and motherhood are not physically attractive and that mothers like themselves less and loathe their bodies more because of them.

If body dissatisfaction has served as a lightning rod for maternal conflict, it's time to stand up and give those responsible a deadly shock.

Six

Manorexia

As a boy growing up in Middle America, I was exposed to the incredible hulks of the day, TV wrestling champions such as Bobo Brazil and Dick the Bruiser. Arnold Schwarzenegger was new on the scene as world body-building champion, winning the Mr Olympia contest seven times, his motivational motto being, 'It's simple; if it jiggles, it's fat'.

I also noticed that many American boys were chunkier than me, so I took up weight lifting and noticed adverts in the back of comic books for what could be described as the antithesis of Slim Fast – 'Weight-On', an ultra-high-calorie flavoured syrup guaranteed to 'put weight on *fast*'. (A woman's worst nightmare!) The sickly-tasting, high-fat, high-sugar concoction didn't make me muscle-bound, nor did it add any meat to my bones. It did, however, give me stomach cramps.

Today, boys and young men are lifting more weights and swallowing far more potent and often dangerous supplements. It isn't only women who want a different body; mixed messages linking physical fitness with body-image insecurities have settled in nicely at home in the male psyche too.

Preventing and dealing with body dissatisfaction and related disorders in men has lagged badly behind that in women. Seeing how men do body dissatisfaction may provide an informative view of how the other half fret and help put your own concerns in perspective.

Big Boy

Body dissatisfaction in men has existed to some extent throughout the ages. During medieval times, in an effort to appear more masculine, muscular and intimidating, men would stuff their shirts with hay or wear bulky armour. Yet despite its long history, male body dissatisfaction remains a profoundly under-recognised (but growing) problem. It also expresses itself very differently from its female equivalent.

The portrayal of men as fat-free and chiselled is dramatically more prevalent than it was a generation ago. While the feminine ideal is thin, the masculine ideal is muscular and 'ripped'. And as with the female market for weight loss, there is the male counterpart to matters of size, with titles such as 'From Geek to Freak: How I Gained 34 lbs. of Muscle in 4 Weeks!' which goes on to describe 'how to triple your testosterone, techniques for producing 15-minute female orgasms, and more.'[1] Then there's the 'Skinny to Muscular Diet' or 'How to Go From Skinny to Muscular in 7 Steps' (with a diet plan). Here's a taste of how:

1. Eat More, Add Calories.
2. Eat 6x a Day.
3. Eat Calorie Dense Food ...[2]

Studies show that while the majority of females studied want to be smaller in size, males are evenly split between those wanting to be bigger (more muscular) versus thinner/more defined with less fat. Younger men are more likely to want to gain weight and the older men to lose weight.[3]

Although body-image issues may not be as common in men as they are with women, they are more prevalent among men than we previously thought and may have damaging consequences.[4] Depression, disordered eating, anxiety, sexual problems, muscle dysmorphia, low self-esteem, compulsive exercise and use of per-formance-enhancing substances have all been directly associated with negative body image in men.[5] And as with women, body dissatisfaction increases the risk of eating disorders, which kill males just as easily.

Body-image concerns are now appearing in boys at much earlier ages than we previously thought.[6] In the same way that women may not be aware of the extent to which their genes and hormones may influence their size, shape and body-fat dis-tribution, boys and young men aren't aware that the ability to gain extra muscle is partly genetic and also limited by age. Testosterone is crucial for gaining muscle size and strength and some males are naturally endowed with higher levels than others, and will therefore have an easier time building their muscles. Testosterone levels peak around the age of thirty, so many males will have to wait or accept their natural limita-tions. But they don't want to wait. And the fitness media and supplement industry fuels their impatience.

Enter the rise of muscle dysmorphia (MDM) – the new-kid-on-the-block male body-image disorder appearing at progressively younger ages. Unlike anorexia nervosa, in which the person wrongly sees him or herself as too big or overweight, the individual with muscle dysmorphia or 'bigorexia' believes that his body is too small and lacking in muscle. Adolescent boys now want to be 14–18kg heavier.[7] And a new study 'Muscle-enhancing Behaviors Among Adolescent Girls and Boys', published by the American Academy of Pediatrics makes for sober reading: 'Boys' body dissatisfaction has simultaneously increased, and research has demonstrated that exposure to images of extremely muscular models contributes to body dissatisfaction and muscle dysmorphia in young men.' Thirty-five per cent of adolescents adopted 'unhealthy muscle-enhancing strategies', including protein powders, steroids and other substances.[8]

Pump It Up

Research with Australian adolescent males[9] found that they do not believe that the mass media influences their body image. But what people say and what they do are often two different things. A study exposing men to controlled images of male bodies found that those who viewed the idealised images of men's bodies actually chose heavier dumbbell weights to lift when performing bicep curls than those who viewed the average images.[10]

The effects of media images start before boys even reach puberty. While attention has been focused on the violent content of computer game imagery, an additional key influence on boys has been operating under the radar. A year-long study, 'Gaming magazines and the drive for muscularity in preadolescent boys', found that those boys who, at the beginning of the year, tended to read mostly gaming magazines reported concerns about their body size at the end of the year, as compared with boys who read fitness and fashion magazines. Sports magazines elicited a similar, but weaker effect – perhaps because their image of masculinity is slightly more realistic.[11] A recent analysis of 'virtual muscularity' – how muscular computer game characters are –

reported that the cyberworld is awash with hypermuscular male characters, and that, ' ... on every dimension measured', male video game characters were 'systematically larger' than the average American male.[12] In effect, boys are being submerged by the opposite of the size-zero images that stoke body dissatisfaction in girls.

The result of this trickle-down effect to the young is now affecting their education. In a survey of its members across the UK, the Association of Teachers and Lecturers found 51 per cent thought boys had low confidence in their body image with 30 per cent reporting that it caused anxiety in male pupils who were then prone to start excessive exercise regimes. This was a main topic in their 2013 annual conference.[13]

The Love Muscle

In the study 'Beyond muscles. Unexplored parts of men's body image' researchers found that while 83 per cent of men wanted to be more muscular, the drive for growth extended beyond their pecs: 68 per cent desired a larger penis (and 62 per cent wanted less body hair).[14] Penis satisfaction, along with its length and girth, is now being measured as part of the examination of overall male body satisfaction. Dissatisfaction with one's penis size correlates with sexual performance anxiety, 'sexual depression and decreased sexual self-esteem' and predicts 'low appearance self-esteem'.[15]

The extent to which body dissatisfaction is leading men to be interested in bigging themselves up down south is staggering and has spawned a whopper of a miracle penis-enlargement market. And to deal with this man-size problem, men buy the books: *Secrets of Penis Size*, *Penis Enlargement that Works* or *The Giant Penis Enlargement Exercise Program*. They take the tablets: 'ULTIMATE-X PENIS ENHANCEMENT/ENLARGE-MENT PILLS 4 Capsules at £14.99!' And when they're not pumping iron they take to the 'Master Gauge Penis Pump. Giving you a bigger length & bigger girth!'

This outbreak of glandular fever mirrors many of the body-part insecurities of women, along with the market exploiting them.

Penis length (and lengthening) is an area of serious research. The *British Journal of Urology International* published a study finding merit in a form of Pilates for the penis. The study, which tested 'the "efficacy" and tolerability of a penile extender device in the treatment of "short penis"' placed the man's penis in traction using the Andropenis device for between four and six hours a day for six months.[16]

As with miracle weight loss and anti-ageing cures, penis pills, creams, brutal stretching exercises, terrifying-looking devices and surgery are all on offer. And almost none of it works. The few approaches that may work often have minimal benefits and serious side effects, including erectile dysfunction. Michael O'Leary, professor of urologic surgery at Harvard Medical School, clears up the matter: 'Trust me, if I knew of a way to safely and effectively increase penis size, I'd be a billionaire. But I don't. Nobody does.'

And as is often the case of women of a healthy weight who insist on dieting because of body dissatisfaction, studies show that most of the men seeking penis enlargement are actually average-sized or above average, but are convinced they're below. Those healthily hung men who can't be convinced otherwise even have a psychiatric diagnosis: penile dysmorphic disorder. It's similar to the distorted perception of anorexics who, no matter how thin they get, are utterly convinced they're fat. The urology journal *BJU International* published a research review of over sixty years' worth of studies entitled,

'Penile size and the "small-penis syndrome"', reporting that actually having a small penis is a relatively rare phenomenon, and small-penis syndrome is much more common in men with normal-sized penises than in those who really do have a small 'micropenis' with a flaccid length of less than 7cm. One study found that 63 per cent of men complaining of small penises said their anxieties started with childhood comparisons and 37 per cent blamed erotic images viewed in their teenage years. None of the men studied actually had a micropenis.[17] Like the slender images of women today, making you feel big and less attractive through unrealistic comparisons, for young impressionable men, Internet porn may be cultivating a rise in penis dissatisfaction.

Wanting to be a big boy is certainly neither new nor Western. A study in the *Asian Journal of Andrology* of 'self-esteem of penile size in young Korean military men' reported that penile augmentation is growing in popularity in Korea and found that soldiers' misjudgment of their own manhood could lead to unjustified surgery.[18]

Willies of the world

The desire for body modification for greater body satisfaction has produced bizarre practices used by men worldwide to enhance the size of their penis. The Topinama of Brazil encourage poisonous snakes to bite their penises to enlarge them for six months, while Indian Sadhu men are reported to use weights to increase the length of theirs and Dayak men in Borneo pierce the head of their penis and insert items into the holes to stimulate their partner.[19]

But men still won't listen to reason or even their perfectly sexually satisfied partners. The study 'Does Size Matter?' involving 55,000 men and women found that although 85 per cent of women were satisfied with their partner's penile size, 45 per cent of men were dissatisfied and wanted to be bigger. Only 0.2 per cent wanted to be smaller.[20]

It's easy to laugh at this state of affairs, and I admit that when I look at this from a distance I do find my gender's penis-comparison mentality ridiculous. Yet those who work in this field justifiably urge caution that men's complaints about the size of their penis are taken seriously. So please forgive me for continuing with the Carry-On tone . . .

Silly Willy

While the penile peer pressure of comparing yourself to others and ending up feeling short-changed is described by some as 'locker-room syndrome', the media have played a role here too. The effects on men of seeing too many well-hung Viagra-fed porno images has a lot in common with the effects of idealised slender images on women. Scientists now suspect that 'women's exaggerated sexual responses to overly endowed men in these pornographic images may also convince men that women have strong preferences for large penises'. Even though most men are perfectly aware at a rational, conscious level that the penises in these pornographic images are unbelievably big, constant exposure may cause them to misjudge the size of their own. The researchers ask, 'Why are so many men dissatisfied with their penis size when the vast majority of women are satisfied with their partner's penis size?'[21] Others offer answers: 'Media marketed to men (pornography, popular magazines) may emphasize the importance of supersized penises, whereas media marketed to women may not.'[22]

Men viewing high levels of Internet pornography may threaten democracy as we know it. As I am writing this chapter the BBC is reporting 'Parliamentary porn consumption laid bare in official figures: more than 300,000 attempts were made to access pornographic websites at the Houses of Parliament in the past year, official records suggest.'[23] Intensive exposure to images of overly endowed men is likely to leave our leaders feeling inadequate. And history tells us how men who feel genitally inadequate behave.

As one form of media feeds body dissatisfaction, another offers gentlemen's relief in the form of conveniently placed adverts which include testimonials reinforcing men's belief that women are more sexually satisfied by larger penises: 'I'm [now] 8 in. and much thicker. My girlfriend wants it all the time.'

Advertisements for surgical enlargement of the penis appear in the sports sections of major newspapers such as the *Los Angeles Times* and include captions like 'Size Matters' and 'Bigger is Better', promising men great benefits to pursuing surgery, such as increased confidence and desirability to women. Advertisers' websites feature before-and-after surgery photos and testimonials, including some from women: 'Since his surgery, he has more confidence. And, to my surprise, I have been overwhelmed with the difference in our sex life. His increased length and especially his added thickness have satisfied me more than I ever dreamed possible.'[24]

And as a phallocentric counterpart to the women's slimming-down book *The Weight Loss Bible* there's now *The Penis Enlargement Bible* '... learn how to get **MASSIVE** growth using only your hands and some readily available natural supplements ...'

And then there's the follow-up book entitled *Larger Than Life*.

The Six-pack

Moving beyond the love muscle, back above the belt, men are increasingly concerned about being hard elsewhere. You may have noticed the obsession in men's magazines with the 'six-pack', accompanied by front-cover photos of ripped, oiled, glistening abdominal muscles and features on core workouts and six-pack secrets promising, '... you'll appear hewn from stone in no time ... shortcuts to earn rock-hard abs fast' and 'a granite midsection'.[25]

The focus is on spending only a few minutes a day, yet getting fast results using photos as testimony. However, even if men do manage to produce rock-hard abdominal muscles, we may never be able to see them as there's often little or no mention of the fact that all the sit-ups in the world will not produce 'spot reduction' of the body fat covering men's stomach muscles. The six-pack look requires an absence of fat hiding the muscles you're trying to put on display which, in turn, requires a change in diet, inheriting the right genes and being of a young age, something you can't buy or train for so easily. Men are left comparing their frontal offerings with the ubiquitous flatter, harder versions presented by the media and thinking, 'I should be able to get one of those too.'

To get that ideal muscular body with that showcase six-pack, men and even school-aged boys have been turning to anabolic steroids – drugs that increase muscle mass, strength and 'hardness' of physique.[26] The head of research and development at the Drug Control Centre, King's College, London recently voiced his concerns about the increasing use of anabolic steroids and the profound effect their marketing is having on young men: 'If you go back twenty years, anabolic-steroid abuse was confined to two groups: one was competitive body

111

builders and the other was athletes who wanted to cheat and improve their performance. Now there is a category, which is young men who take anabolic steroids for cosmetic reasons.'[27] In England, a growing number of young Asians are using steroids to try and build up muscle and achieve the perfect body, according to drugs workers. For example, needle-exchange centres in Luton report that 84 per cent of Asians visiting them take steroids.[28]

In addition to its 'body-bulking' properties, a secondary effect of the steroid is to burn fat to reveal those muscles. But for many, taking 'cutting steroids' isn't enough and they add human growth hormone, and even bronchial medication or thyroid medication to increase the amounts of fat lost. In the past few years a range of new, but untested drugs has emerged, as marketers keep one step ahead of the health and legal authorities.[29] An Australian study, not yet published, of boys from twenty-eight state and private high schools found more than a quarter of fifteen- to seventeen-year-olds reported having used sports supplements, vitamins or minerals to gain weight and muscle. And a significant number reported using medication or drugs, such as steroids, insulin injections and 'muscle-building pills'.[30]

It seems you can't reason with many men, who look at their bodies in the mirror and then take their steroids, despite the clear sobering warnings of shrinkage of the testicles (testicular atrophy), reduced sperm count or infertility, baldness, development of breasts (gynaecomastia) and an increased risk of prostate cancer.[31]

Some young men and schoolboys even die in the pursuit of the six-pack as a result of taking steroids. In raising awareness about the dangers of APEDs (Appearance & Performance Enhancing Drugs), the founder of the Matthew Dear Foundation in the UK draws a useful comparison in body dissatisfaction: 'Society is very aware of girls wanting to be like models, wanting to be stick-thin and taking diet pills, but we are not aware of the pressures put on young men to be like their role models, look a certain way, to have a certain image. They have got to have the six-pack and the rippling muscles.'[32]

But in the way that women's weight and dress size have suffered from deflation down towards a size zero, the six-pack too is now being rendered passé by the rise of the new look, as *Men's Health* entices men to 'Build an eight-pack in less time' with no-fuss exercises which 'are 100% more useful than lying on the floor and grunting'.[33]

Whether striving for a six- or eight-pack, males are pursuing something socially acceptable at a time when the industrialised world is up in arms about obesity. Yet this backdrop may conceal the body dissatisfaction and eating disorders that underlie an impressive 200 sit-ups a day. Instead of using food as a voice for expressing unhappiness or pain, men can eat normally yet over-exercise, thereby burning too many calories, and take 'cutting steroids' or other products such as 'thermogenic fat strippers', which mask what is, in effect, an eating disorder. And in the same way that permarexic women may receive tacit approval for their slight look, the cut, over-lean sharply defined bodies of men may elicit social approval at a time of sloth and nutritional plenty.

After all, exercise is deemed good and so are six-packs.

Cutting Comments

Weight- and shape-based, appearance-related comments have been shown to negatively affect the mental health and wellbeing of women in a well-documented body of research. And the same effect is now showing up in studies of men. In a novel study published in *Psychology of Men & Masculinity* men who received positive comments were more likely to experience less body dissatisfaction, but then go ahead and do more of what caused them to receive the positive comments to begin with – muscle building. Men who reported receiving more negative comments were more likely to have higher body dissatisfaction and disordered eating.[34]

The New Man in the Mirror

Beyond men's preoccupation with the size and shape of their bodies, something that I would have thought unthinkable is happening: even the most unlikely beasts can now be found moisturising and waxing. The latest 'Face Moisturizer Manufacturing Market Research Report' concludes that men's skincare products have become a noteworthy group, estimating that male-centred care items account for about one-third of the industry.[35]

At the gym I've heard tough, tattoo-covered, blue-collar men discuss, compare and contrast the merits and demerits of various methods of hair removal, swapping stories about how their last waxing session made them wince with pain.

And so it doesn't look as if men's increasing body awareness is going to subside in the near future. However, there are still great examples of more traditional expressions of male body image.

Belly Barging

For men, size will always matter. As a final point of comparison, it's worth mentioning how some men express their body image in a more colourful way, wearing their protruding stomachs with great pride and putting their bulging bellies to good use – in belly barging.

The sport of gut barging involves two abdominally well-endowed men greasing their bellies up with engine oil, which helps to create a great slapping sound as the two fat men ram each other belly-to-belly in an attempt to push each other off the belly-barging mat. The spectacular rise in paunch power was even showcased at the Royal Albert Hall in London. Binky Braithwaite has been referred to as the 'Gutfather' of belly barging after moving on from his career as the leader of CAMDA (the Campaign to Abolish Morris Dancing Absolutely). He turned to the belly to reposition the modern male image after seeing Morris dancing in pubs as 'the biggest threat to our wellbeing. Morris men, with beards ... start namby-pambying outside the country pub where you are having a quiet drink. Now, apparently, they are to be financed by the National Lottery. Is this the sort of country we want?'

In 1996 when the art form was just emerging, the *Independent* newspaper reported attempts by the British belly bargers to entice their Japanese sumo wrestling counterparts over. The President of the World Gut-barging Association offered 'the hand of friendship to our larger Japanese cousins ... to embrace them warmly into the bosom of the gut-barging family. We cannot offer fish and boiled rice, but we can keep them in fighting condition on our diet of British beef, bulls' semen and deep-fried Mars bars.'

I can't imagine women strutting their over-stuffed stuff in this way, nor seeking such abdominal accolades, but it certainly is a very different way to think about body image.

PART TWO

The Shape Of Things To Come

Unlike other forms of contamination or health risk such as air pollution or sugar or passive smoke, the causes of body dissatisfaction are difficult to identify and reduce simply. And unlike preventing sunburn, whereby strong sunlight can be blocked with the right SPF screen, covering up or by stepping into the shade, the rays of body images don't travel in a straight line, often come from your own mind and are more difficult to simply block.

It's clear that the factors that influence the way you feel about your body are widespread, often involving things that are abstract or cultural: 'probably the result of some "socially transmitted" standard of "ideal" body image'.[1] We need changes from the top down; however, we can't afford to wait for this to happen, so in the meantime we need to adjust our own lives in a way that will indirectly and directly improve body dissatisfaction. It would be unethical to suggest that there is a quick self-help fix to banish body dissatisfaction, enabling you to learn to absolutely 'love your body' – and to do so would, frankly, sound exactly like the self-improvement promises splashed across the front cover of the very magazines that have helped cause body dissatisfaction in the first place.

However, as with many problems, the effects can be lessened significantly, enabling us to lead less troubled, healthier and more fulfilling lives. So while you may ultimately never be elated at the thought of stepping on the scales naked in front of the mirror, there is a great deal of wiggle room to be had in terms of making you feel more comfortable with your size and shape. And in the case of young girls, there's much we can do to prevent them from suffering body dissatisfaction the way their predecessors have.

Most women do not have body dissatisfaction to the extent that it is a clinical problem requiring psychiatric intervention, and the following chapters are intended for this vast majority who experience this 'normative discontent' (see p. 3). From a practical point of view, if at least half of all females are experiencing body dissatisfaction, there wouldn't be enough therapists to go around, and while it may seem difficult to know the hazy dividing line between 'normal' and severe body dissatisfaction requiring expert help, there are some ways of distinguishing. There is some further information in the Resources section (see p. 247) to help you answer this question.

A Model of Body Image Resilience

Despite the ubiquitous pressures on women to have a slim-and-beautiful appearance, there is a subset who do actually feel satisfied with their bodies and do not face problems in this area of the lives. Their perceptions and experiences can offer valuable information about protective factors that might buffer others against body dissatisfaction. How do some women manage to resist the strong sociocultural pressures that might otherwise sway them to be dissatisfied with their bodies?

As science closes in on the actual causes and mechanisms behind body dissatisfaction, some researchers have shifted their focus to understanding and cultivating 'resilience' in the face of body-image pressures. A great deal of progress is now being made in identifying and harnessing systems for the protection of young women against the development of body dissatisfaction and related maladaptive eating, while helping to enhance their body image. This area of work is referred to as a 'Body-image Resilience Model'. For example, research by the Universities of Arizona and Louisiana 'identified protective factors that may promote body satisfaction', including 'family social support, understanding today's sociocultural pressure, actively rejecting of the "superwoman ideal", active coping and wellness.'[2]

There are some countermeasures we can take – for you as an individual woman, and for parents, schools and government as well – that in concert, over time, can have a very positive effect on the way people feel about their bodies and, therefore, about their self-worth. Our approach to most psychological issues is increasingly preoccupied with applying a 'technique' that cures the problem. We often assume that anything that is effective has been organised, has a label and is usually commodified, packaged and for sale. After all, why would anyone want to promote something that is readily accessible and subtle at a time when branding (even of psychological therapies), product placement and 'partnership deals' enable self-improvement to be rendered profitable? Yet many of the measures I'm about to outline may at first seem downright ordinary, freely available and most definitely not 'technique-based'. And it is no coincidence that they have no manufacturer, lobby group, media or financial base.

Seven

Paradigm Shift

Few of us travel through life luggage-free; most of us have baggage, and in many instances it contains our somewhat tattered body image. But something that's becoming clear is that involving ourselves in areas of life that engage us, providing a sense of control, competence and accomplishment, works strongly in favour of increased body satisfaction. This is partly a consequence of putting the eggs of our self-esteem in a variety of baskets. Put simply, if we are engaged and invested in other things, we simply have less room and time for feeling or thinking about our bodies.

This is not a form of denial or evasion, but a necessary redistribution of our emotional and intellectual resources to a more realistic balance – a correction in our attention economy ensuring we pay attention to a more deserving and widely spread range of things in our lives.

In fact, being preoccupied with and distressed about your body may be serving as an avoidance of more difficult life issues that you face. Focusing on your body and trying to change it may give you greater *perception* of control, along with the illusion that changing your body will change your life. These behaviours keep you from learning that attractiveness is not the sole determining factor in happiness and success. It can also lead to social isolation.

Painful Lessons

One way to think of body dissatisfaction is as an underlying, low-level, often subliminal, yet ever-present discomfort, distress or pain. Pain can be reduced by shifting attention to something else, so robbing the source of pain of our full attentional resources. For instance, you have lower-back pain; yet while you're engrossed in a book or film the pain is less prominent or even goes unnoticed.

We can learn a few lessons by looking at cognitive methods of reducing physical discomfort by altering our awareness, perception, reasoning and judgment to our advantage. In evaluating 'psychological interventions for reducing pain and distress during routine childhood immunisations' researchers found that distraction provided by either the child, nurse or parent was effective in reducing pain and/or distress.[1] And pain relief through distraction is not all in your mind. Studies using high-resolution spinal fMRI (functional magnetic resonance imaging) show that mental distractions actually inhibit the physiological response to incoming pain signals at the earliest stage, reducing the number of pain signals travelling up from the spinal cord to higher-order brain regions that would normally tell you that you hurt.

Another example of shifting our focus to reduce discomfort is listening to music. Researchers from the University of Utah Pain Research Center evaluated the potential benefits of music for diverting our psychological responses to experimental pain – electric shocks administered by the scientists. They think music may divert our cognitive focus from pain by providing intellectual and emotional engagement. Interestingly, those people with high levels of anxiety about pain had the greatest engagement with the music.[2] Another study involving children undergoing painful medical procedures in a hospital Accident and Emergency department also found that music may have a positive impact on pain and distress.[3]

Distraction in a more general sense may be a good way to take your mind off your body which is a good policy for dealing with body dissatisfaction.

Attentional Body Bias

People with greater body dissatisfaction are often described as having an 'attentional bias' – being more 'self-focused'. They are more aware of their body's appearance, instead of focusing on what they see around them or on what they're currently doing. This, in turn, reinforces their over-awareness of their appearance and maintains a cycle. In trying to change this attentional bias some clinicians ask people to first monitor where their attention is being focused:

- On you – e.g. assessing your appearance to other people or how you feel.
- On what you're doing – e.g. a conversation or a task you're engaged in.
- On your surroundings – sounds of birds or traffic in the background.

With more body dissatisfaction you are likely to focus the greater proportion of your attention on yourself, and the goal of therapy or self-help is to teach you to focus more on what you're doing and on your surroundings.[4]

Shifting attention away from your body and how it looks may come across as too simplistic, but attention – the act or faculty of applying one's mind – is the prerequisite to experience. Attention is the focus control on your lens that looks out on life; it is a defining requirement for what we consider being alive. So whether you want to recite Proust, order a pizza or slap someone in the face, you have to be able to pay attention to things in order to experience them. Some scientists now suspect that a failure in our ability to control attention and to therefore fully engage with our surroundings can cause boredom which, in turn, may lead to depression. For example, we may go to a concert expecting a stimulating, enjoyable evening of music, yet an inability to focus our attention on it drains all colour from the event. This lack of immersion in the world beyond our own thoughts could lead us to evaluate our experiences as meaningless, which is not very happy-making.[5]

The Attention Economy

Attention may be something we take for granted, but capitalist boardrooms and the advertising industry are certainly on to it. The *Harvard Business Review* and Harvard Business School Press publish articles and entire books on the 'attention economy'. Observations within the book entitled *The Attention Economy* include business mantras such as, 'Like airplane seats and fresh food, attention is a highly perishable commodity', and ' ... there's a cash market for human attention, the most coveted commodity of all'. Or, as one ad man once put it: 'The money's where the eyeballs are.' I've always felt that naked capitalism is a most revealing scientific method, in that it is willing to recognise anything that will make a profit. So take it from Wall Street: pay attention to attention.

I'm not trying to be insensitive, but simply focusing away from the *self* can be very positive, both for us and others too. Our society has brought about a paramountcy of the self, blurring the distinction between reasonable concepts of self-respect, self-esteem, self-awareness and self-reflection ... and self-absorption, along with its relative – being self-conscious. An interesting aspect of this was revealed in a study by the University of Queensland School of Population Health involving young adults who have moved away from traditional religious beliefs towards more self-focused religions and spirituality, and who were shown to be up to twice as likely to feel anxious and depressed. Lead author Dr Rosemary Aird said that most non-religious forms of spirituality were too individualistic: 'Their focus on self-fulfilment and self-improvement and the lack of emphasis on others' wellbeing appears to have the potential to undermine a person's mental health and social relationships ... The New Spirituality promotes the idea that self-transformation will lead to a positive and constructive change in self and society. But there is a contradiction – how can one change society in a positive way if one is primarily focused on oneself?'[6]

Once you do begin to shift attention away from your body image and even your self, *where* you refocus your attention matters too.

Preventing or coping with body dissatisfaction is often less a case of actively doing and saying positive things or 'celebrating' our bodies, and more a case of reducing negative things. If anything, bodies should be thought about less and merely taken for granted. We may not be able to control many of the influences that cause body dissatisfaction, but we can opt to lead our lives in ways that work around them or walk straight over them: we

127

can do things, go places and interact with people that work against body dissatisfaction.

Pay attention to Mother Nature

One thing many of us overlook or take for granted is the benefit of being outdoors in nature. However, the medical establishment is now recognising the psychological and physical health benefits. As a general step in shifting our focus away from our bodies, spending more time in a green environment may improve our ability to direct our attention to where we want it and may also generally improve our mental health and even self-esteem.[7]

A growing number of researchers now believe that being exposed to greenery has general benefits for our ability to pay attention. Studies refer to 'superior attentional functioning' and the fact that 'the effect of nature on inattention is robust'. A study published in the *American Journal of Public Health* found that exposing children with attention deficit hyperactivity disorder (ADHD) to outdoor greenery was strongly associated with a reduction in their symptoms. And the greener the setting, the greater the reduction in symptoms. In a follow-up study children with ADHD were taken on twenty-minute walks in one of three environments – a city park and two other well-kept urban settings. The benefits were substantial and considered comparable to those reported for ADHD prescription medicines. They concluded that spending twenty minutes in a green park setting was sufficient to improve attention, compared to spending the same amount of time in other settings 'for all income groups and for both boys and girls'.

The investigators also pointed to research conducted among people without ADHD, showing that inattention and impulsivity are reduced after exposure to green natural views and settings.[8]

It's also thought that nature buffers the impact of life's stresses on children and helps them deal with adversity: the greater the amount of nature exposure, the greater the benefits.[9]

The intriguing paper 'Can Nature Make Us More Caring?' raises the question of whether exposure to more greenery can influence our orientation away from focusing on ourselves to focusing on others. The research showed that young people 'immersed in natural environments' expressed greater generosity and concern for others than those immersed in 'non-natural environments'.[10] And you'll see later, caring for others can be hugely beneficial not only for those on the receiving end, but for you too.

Other research has suggested that green environments may reduce anxiety, and reduced anxiety could, in turn, improve athletic performance. Research also shows that plants have psychological and restorative value, such as improving coping mechanisms in human subjects, as well as the potential to increase concentration and focus attention that could affect performance of athletes. A research team at the University of Texas investigated the impact of greenery/landscaping on athletic performance and emotional and physical anxiety in track and field athletes and found that the level of greenness was a predictor of the best performance by the athletes. More of the athletes' best performance marks were at the track and field site that had the highest greenery rating, while many of their worst were at those with the lowest greenery rating.[11]

Plus, even small doses of outdoor physical activity for as little as five minutes at a time may have significant effects on our mental health. There is growing evidence that 'green exercise' – combining activities such as walking or cycling in nature – boosts wellbeing more than just exercise alone. A recent study by the Department of Biological Sciences, University of Essex found, 'Every green environment improved both self-esteem and mood'. *All* types of green physical activity led to improvements in measures of mental health and, most surprising to the researchers was that the strongest response was seen almost immediately. 'This study confirms that the environment provides an important health service.'[12] And, of course, improved self-esteem provides greater protection against body dissatisfaction.

Lastly, research involving over 10,000 people by the European Centre for Environment & Human Health, University of Exeter Medical School found that people reported less mental distress and higher life satisfaction when they were living in greener areas. This held true even after the researchers accounted for differences in income, employment, marital status, physical health and housing.[13] This may not seem directly related to making you love your body, but the general background mental benefits of more green time can give you a quiet resilience in the face of body dissatisfaction.

Attentional restoration

But how can something as mundane as a tree or a flowerbed or grass exert any biological and cognitive effects on people? One main area of interest is the possibility that our attentional system becomes overworked and tired and the effect of nature may help remedy this, thereby improving our ability to pay sustained attention.

Modern life is geared toward 'multitasking' and distraction, with our attention tantalised and then submerged under a tyranny of options. Just consider the modern home with an average of five or more TV, computer and other screens and smartphones – described as an ecosystem of interruption technologies. Paying sustained attention with full engagement is not easy when our culture and economy wants it diverted to all the exciting things on offer.

Interestingly, new findings suggest that people living in an urbanised environment – which is the majority of people in the developed world – are not functioning at their optimum level of attentional engagement. Scientists examined the effect of urbanisation on a remote Namibian tribe and found that those who had not moved to an urbanised environment were more able to concentrate in cognitive tests. The researchers suggested that urban environments 'prioritise distraction' by exploring all the stimulation on offer 'at the expense of attentional engagement and cognitive control of attentional selection'.[14]

When your attentional system becomes tired, greenery is thought to provide 'attentional restoration'. The explanations seem to revolve around the way greenery effortlessly engages our attention, allowing us to attend without paying attention. The information-processing demands of everyday life, including electronic media, mobile telephones, increasing consumer and 'lifestyle choices' and associated decisions – take their toll on our intellectual and emotional resources. We increasingly shift attention between various things – multitasking – and are encouraged to do so. This modern life causes a temporary 'attention fatigue' which may be corrected when our underlying attention system has an opportunity to rest. And natural green environments are thought to help in this because they engage our minds effortlessly. So the sense of rejuvenation we often experience after spending time in natural settings may, in part, reflect a 'recharging' of some parts of our attentional system.

An intriguing article in the *Lancet* – 'Green space, psychological restoration, and telomere length' – suggests a possible longer-term influence of green environments on our DNA and chromosomes that may have restorative benefits and also affect our rate of ageing: 'The results show that the presence of green spaces could have health benefits in terms of biological ageing ... We therefore agree that the psychological benefit arising from a restorative environment could be a real one.'[15]

We are hard-wired to gravitate toward greenery. Our ancestors who sought green areas or lived as subsistence hunters, gatherers and farmers were more likely to eat, drink and survive. Today, many of the benefits associated with our exposure to greenery may be part of an evolutionary reward system reinforcing the very thing that kept us alive for hundreds of thousands of years.

An RDA for greenery?

A recent series of studies at the University of Rochester in the US had particularly robust findings that being outside in green nature for just twenty minutes in a day was enough to significantly boost vitality levels. Professor of psychiatry Richard Ryan, the lead author, commented, 'Nature is fuel for the soul'.[16] So surely a conservative minimum average of twenty minutes' exposure to greenery a day is a very reasonable investment.

Biologists have recently pointed to a fundamental shift away from an appreciation of nature – 'biophilia' – to 'videophilia', a focus on sedentary activities involving electronic media.[17] Aside from displacing time that they believe could have been spent outdoors exposed to greenery, videophilia also exposes us to a great number of idealised slender body images. When you think that people stare at an indoor television screen for thirty hours a week, with all the effects this may entail, using some of those hours to expose yourself to greenery – something that is more likely to make you feel better about yourself – is certainly worth the effort.

It's a shame to think that we live in a time when scientific evidence has to be provided in favour of something our grand-parents took for granted. Still, stressing the need for more exposure to something we enjoy anyway, but never considered a health practice is nice for a change.

Locus of Control

Trying to lead our lives in a way that bolsters our sense of influence over our selves and our lives may create a more resilient backdrop, making it more difficult for body dissatisfaction to flourish. The concept of 'locus of control' refers to our general belief that what happens to us is mainly either under *our own* control (internal locus) or a matter of chance or *outside* controllable factors (external locus). While our degree of internal/external locus of control may be powerfully influenced by behavioural genetics, along with our upbringing and earlier life experiences, it is still affected by our subsequent experiences.[18] Studies of children and adults in a variety of settings have reported shifts in people's locus of control brought about by various approaches.

For example, teaching students a skill that increases their sense of control over something – even a skill as unusual as controlling their own finger temperature – was found to enhance their general sense of control over wider events. A laboratory-based study of young adults found that biofeedback-assisted autogenic training (controlling your own finger temperature) seemed to make them 'significantly more internal in their locus of control after training'.[19]

It seems that by learning to control things in a 'hands-on' context, people may gain a more general sense of control over other areas of their lives. Some refer to this as 'mastery experiences'.

In clinical studies, increased internal locus of control has been found to have a lower association with suffering from anxiety and a reduced risk of suffering from depression, other psychological disorders and behavioural problems.[20]

Even something medical and physiological, such as the level of insulin resistance in diabetic patients, is significantly lower in those who have a higher internal locus of control.[21] And learning about their condition in a group as opposed to an individual setting was also found to increase patients' internal locus of control.

Survivors of natural disasters have shown considerable benefit from craft-based activities which seem to work as 'diversional therapy', as well as giving the individual a sense of control over what they are doing, which may have a general effect of increasing their internal locus of control. This 'diversional therapy' has become an integral part of the Red Cross's regional development.[22]

Locus of control is now also of interest in reducing teenage violence and aggression. Teenagers who believe in the idea that individuals can change are likely to have an 'internal locus of control' and consider that their actions have an influence on their current and future activities and those of others. Investigators from the University of Texas and Stanford University discovered that by educating individuals on the notion that people have the potential to change, aggressive reactions can be reduced.[23] Meanwhile, at the other end of the age spectrum, internal locus of control was found, through cognitive training, to improve even among people over sixty-five, according to a study in the *Journals of Gerontology*.[24]

While locus of control seems an abstract concept, there are some practical implications for body dissatisfaction: by investing ourselves in things that give us a sense of satisfaction and competence, we not only shift our attention away from body issues, but we may also gain a more general sense of influence over our lives, making us more resilient in the face of cultural pressures and even our own personal histories. A general sense of competency emerges.

Eight

Running Away from Body Dissatisfaction

Few people are aware that being physically active is the single most important thing that most of us can do to improve or maintain our health. It not only reduces the risk of developing or dying from cardiovascular disease and diabetes, but also improves mood, builds bones, strengthens muscles, expands lung capacity, reduces the risk of falls and fractures and helps to improve body composition. What's more, physical activity enhances the immune system's ability to detect and fend off certain types of cancer and it also prevents certain cancers. Beyond this, there are also positive changes that occur at the level of cells and molecules for specific conditions such as atherosclerosis and diabetes.

Compared with the well-researched and understood physical benefits of exercise, the psychological benefits have been explored far less. Over the past few years, however, research has added to the menu of benefits to now offer intellectual and psychological perks.

Exercise appears to increase our intellectual capabilities –

specifically the ability to carry out tasks that require attention, organisation and planning. For example, even in older adults, a large analysis by the University of Otago, New Zealand consistently found that fitter people scored better in mental tests than their unfit peers. Additional studies found that scores in mental tests improved in those who were assigned to an aerobic exercise regime compared to stretch and tone classes.[1]

In their report 'Understanding Depression' Harvard Medical School describes research finding that a programme of exercise can be just as effective as antidepressants for people with mild to moderate depression; also that its effects lasted longer than those of antidepressants and that patients were less likely to relapse.[2] Researchers have also found that in people with schizophrenia, exercise programmes improved their mental state including anxiety and depression, particularly when compared to standard care.[3]

The role of physical exercise in promoting mental health may partly involve the release of opioids in our brains – compounds that have similar actions to opiates such as heroin or morphine – in response to exercise, hence the 'opioid theory' of the 'runner's high'.[4] Opioids reduce pain, bring about feelings of wellbeing and improve mood, which may contribute to better mental health. And there's also the 'marijuana prescription for exercise' based on the discovery of endocannabinoids – compounds found in cannabis that our bodies produce naturally in various amounts according to how intensively we exercise.[5] Another theory is that exercise stimulates the neurotransmitter norepinephrine, which may directly improve mood.[6] Either way, the good thing about physical activity is that it can make us feel better in 20–30 minutes and it's generally free.

It's therefore not surprising that in 2013, to highlight Mental Health Awareness Week, Britain's Mental Health Foundation launched a campaign and issued a report 'Let's get Physical'.

'Evidence shows that physical activity is significantly beneficial for people's mental health and wellbeing:

- Even small increases in levels of activity can improve wellbeing and reduce stress levels.
- It can lead to improved body-image, self-esteem and self-worth, as well as providing opportunities for social contact and social interaction.
- Physical activity can act as both prevention and treatment for various mental illnesses including depression and anxiety.'[7]

There are similar moves around the world. For example, the state government of Victoria, Australia advises that regular physical activity helps improve mental health,[8] while Beijing hosted the '1st China Conference of Physical Exercise and Mental Health'. And the mental-health charity Mind has even launched a campaign and issued a statement on the key role of exercise in mental health.[9]

But what actually accounts for the association between exercise and mental health?

A study of 7000 Dutch students examined two existing explanations for the link: either that physical activity has positive effects on body weight and body structure, leading to positive feedback from your peers and improved self-image, ultimately improving mental health; or that the social aspects of physical activity – such as social relationships and mutual support among team members – contribute to the positive links between exercise and mental health. They found that both 'psychosocial' factors – body image and social interaction – were relevant in helping to explain part of the connection between physical activity and mental health. The researchers acknowledge that other factors, such as the physiological effects of exercise mentioned above, are probably also at work.[10]

Others believe that through exercise you can have 'mastery experiences', whereby physical activity can lead to greater feelings of mastery, or the belief that you are able to influence your environment and bring about desired outcomes which, in turn, leads to greater wellbeing. This ties in with the concept of locus of control mentioned elsewhere (see pp. 133–124).

There are also delayed benefits from exercise in young and old with one research team reporting 'a significant lagged effect of physical activity on self-esteem'. Specifically, higher physical activity at ages nine and eleven years predicted higher self-esteem at ages eleven and thirteen years respectively. They found that positive effects of physical activity on self-esteem were most apparent for girls with a higher BMI.[11] In adults aged sixty years and older, other scientists found a direct link between physical activity and increased self-esteem over time. Physical activity appeared to have a positive effect on physical self-worth and global self-esteem over a four-year period.[12]

Exercise and Body Dissatisfaction

Having said that, people who report high body dissatisfaction tend to exercise the least, and so scientists wanted to take it a step further and see whether exercise may cause body image to improve. A systematic analysis of fifty-seven studies of the 'Effects of Exercise Interventions on Body Image' found that exercise markedly improved the way people felt about their bodies, regardless of the actual physical benefits they may derive from it.[13] In fact, exercise improved body image for both fit and unfit alike. And it was the simple act of exercise and not the fitness itself that was thought responsible. People who don't achieve exercise milestones such as losing fat, gaining strength or boosting cardiovascular fitness were found to feel just as good about their bodies as their more athletic counterparts.

In the book *Exercise and Changes in Body Image* the authors examined three meta-analyses on a very large number of studies on this issue. They found that even with the great variety among the studies, the results of every meta-analysis were consistent. Exercise was found to have significant positive effects on body image.[14]

A study on teenagers instructed to exercise twice weekly reported that 'significant pre-post improvements were found for body image, perceived scholastic competence and social competence'. Interestingly, 'these psychological benefits were related to improved aerobic fitness but not changes in body composition.' So even without fat loss, body image improved in relation to the physical exercise alone.[15]

The intensity of the activity also seems to be of importance, as moderate and strenuous exercise have been linked with greater effects on body dissatisfaction than mild-intensity activities.[16] However, it's thought that the amount of exertion required to derive the psychological benefits of exercise, including those relating to body image, may be substantially lower than the amount required to gain the physical benefits.

Pregnancy, Body Dissatisfaction, Mood and Exercise

The problem of body dissatisfaction and mood during pregnancy discussed in Chapter 5, 'Baby Dissatisfaction', is now of increasing interest to exercise researchers.

Women who exercise more prior to their pregnancy are found to have greater body satisfaction during the second and third trimesters and fewer depressive symptoms in the second trimester. It's thought that avid pre-pregnancy exercise might protect women from negative depressive symptoms and body dissatisfaction during mid-to-late pregnancy.

Interestingly, women with greater depressive symptoms during the first trimester tended to engage in less exercise in early pregnancy.[17] 'Roughly 70 per cent of women are inactive during pregnancy ... preliminary research suggests that women who are more physically active during pregnancy report greater body image satisfaction than those who are less active.'[18] While exercise may help to control changes in body fat and weight that could, in turn, influence body satisfaction, there may also be other effects: physical activity may reduce anxiety about bodily changes during pregnancy and may also help sustain a woman's perceptions of her physical competence and self-efficacy.[19]

The American College of Sports Medicine recommends that healthy pregnant women without obstetric complications engage in thirty minutes of moderate exercise most, if not all, days of the week.

Underrated Elixir

It seems that doing virtually any type of exercise on a regular basis can help us feel better about our bodies. People often expect solutions to problems to be complex, long-winded and expensive. Yet the approaches that are quick, simple and free are often the most effective – even without a lobby group or corporate backer behind them.

Physical activity will not solve all of your emotional problems, nor is it a mass panacea for body dissatisfaction. Nevertheless, it's encouraging to know that even short, frequent bouts of lower-intensity exercise can improve our body image. Given that, for example, only 29 per cent of women in England meet the

Chief Medical Officer's bare minimal recommended levels of physical activity, there may be plenty of wiggle room for an improvement in body dissatisfaction by simply being a bit more active.[20] And all of the mental and physical bonuses previously described will also be part of the package deal.

However, as mentioned above and in Chapter 1, 'Size Matters', while exercise may improve body satisfaction, body dissatisfaction can act as a barrier to participating in physical activity in the first place. With this in mind, the Mental Health Foundation advises that attending a female-only exercise class or a ladies-only swimming session may help some women to overcome any anxiety that may be presenting a barrier to exercise. 'Exercising with a companion can also help to reduce social physique anxiety and may be particularly helpful during the first few exercise sessions. The environment can influence how one feels too; gyms with mirrored walls tend to heighten anxiety, as does exercising near a window or other space where one feels "on show".'[21]

Reclaiming 'Exercise'

In his line '*Roga bonam mentem, bonam valitudinem animi, deinde tunc corporis*' ('Exercise promotes a good mind, good spiritual health, finally, health of body'), the Roman philosopher Seneca encapsulated how exercise has been traditionally viewed. Romans sought the benefits sports conferred: 'recreational, health-promoting, or military usefulness'. Romans were practical. The first permanent stadium for athletics wasn't constructed until Domitian (81–96AD), but athletic activity doesn't necessitate a purpose-built location. In addition to the rivers and paths for bathing and staying fit, the public used the baths for games and exercise.[22] If he were alive today observing modern Italians 'going for the burn' in loud crowded mirrored enclosures, Seneca would be spitting chariots.

Around the world when I visit a gym I invariably see pink-faced women being goaded by a personal trainer, helping them to absolve themselves for last night's piece of chocolate cake. In some gyms there is a body-fat analyser on public display to check your progress or otherwise. And there are also large TV monitors on the wall which transmit your name and current workout status (heart rate/calories burning) for all to see. And then there are also smartphone apps, you can check any time, any place.

And so we must also take the values of the gym, health club, leisure centre or class into consideration before inadvertently signing up to more body dissatisfaction and paying for the pleasure. Some places are obsessed with burning calories and body fat – the way you hope to *look* – as opposed to simply improving your health, with appearance being an added bonus. Many of the aerobics, 'hip-and-thigh', 'bums-and-tums', 'calorie-blaster' and the self-loathingly named 'body-combat' classes and DVDs are taught by negative role models who seem infatuated with the goal of banishing female body fat along with your body image. There have been claims and some studies reporting that many of the ultra-fit-and-toned fitness-class instructors have body-image problems and disordered eating themselves.[23] Some experts within the fitness class world remind fitness-class instructors that 'our influence is so strong that we have an obligation to help participants – and our colleagues – have a healthy outlook on their bodies'.[24]

Fitness instructors themselves are under pressure as a result of the hyped stories of celebrities who appear to have transformed their bodies with the help of a particular new exercise regime, designed and imposed by their soon-to-be famous personal trainer who then goes on to make DVDs and appear on breakfast television in a skimpy leotard. This celebrity invasion of what was the timeless, unaffected world of physical activity has caused a corruption of what exercise should be, turning it into a time-consuming regime that most mortals cannot possibly adhere to, with a primary focus on low-fat looks, not on general fitness, health and wellbeing. Physical activity has to be reclaimed by the rest of us who don't have in-house personal trainers and vegan chefs.

Exercising with the explicit intention of speeding up the weight-loss process and as a primary strategy for altering body shape and attractiveness has been associated with increased body dissatisfaction and disordered eating. Meanwhile, functional reasons for exercise such as health, fitness or enjoyment have been linked to increased self-esteem, body esteem and lower levels of body dissatisfaction.

Sensible Seneca

Lack of time is a very common barrier to people taking up physical activity. However, it doesn't have to involve a two-hour trip to a gym or leisure centre. It can be built into your normal life by, for example, walking for short trips, rather than using your car or the bus, walking up stairs, rather than taking the lift or escalator. Some naturally physical activities in your home, such as housework and gardening, are also considered moderate-intensity physical activity, depending on how vigorously you're doing them. And then, of course, there's the great exercise of simply walking your dog.

Our personalities may have some bearing on the type of physical activity we prefer. Someone who likes routine might like a regular, structured exercise regime such as running, whereas a person who likes novelty and gets bored easily might prefer something with more variety, such as circuit training or dance. Some of us like team or group activities, while others prefer to go it alone.

The most important thing is that you feel able to start being more physically active, regardless of the duration or intensity of the physical activity in the first instance. Having choice and control over said activity (the type, frequency and intensity) is more likely to ensure you'll keep doing it and enjoy it more. In addition, gaining a sense of competence as a result of physical activity enhances motivation, as does the fact that it offers the opportunity for meaningful relationships with other people – the same principle that works for bingo and bridge clubs.

If you are currently a couch potato, look at it this way: the biggest health benefits and feel-good factor go to people like you who are beginning from scratch or from a lapsed position and who start to do *some* physical activity, even if it's below the minimum guidelines. So the most important thing is to get started at a level which feels comfortable and build up the duration and intensity of physical activity gradually. For example, a ten-minute brisk walk every day is one simple way to get going, or by building your shopping or some other errand into that walk.

Physical activity is something we can start doing almost immediately to improve body dissatisfaction. And so the Mental Health Foundation puts it well: we need to see 'physical activity as a fundamental and desirable part of our daily lives, not an add-on'.[25]

Nine

Well Connected?

In his book *Modern Man in Search of a Soul* the psychiatrist Carl Jung wrote: 'The meeting of two personalities is like the contact of two chemical substances: if there is any reaction, both are transformed.'[1] While they can, of course, be transformed for the worse, relationships and a sense of connection between people both individually and as a group are vital. It may seem mechanistic to describe our relationships and connections in terms of being a 'medical necessity', but that is precisely what new research is finding. People need people – probably because we evolved and survived by interacting and forming bonds and social groups. Jung would be pleased to know that when people meet there does literally seem to be a chemical reaction.

Chemistry of Connection

Although the relationship between social support and body dis-satisfaction remains unclear and complex, within families there is some evidence that social support can help with the phenomenon.[2] It is generally thought to provide significant mental and physical health benefits and to be a great source of resilience in the face of insecurity and adversity. For example, in pointing out 'protective factors' that work against the development of eating disorders, Australia's Department of Health's National Eating Disorders Collaboration cites 'family connectedness' and 'eating regular meals with the family', while conceding that it helps by 'belonging to a family that does not overemphasise weight and physical attractiveness'.[3] Social support is considered a buffer against life stressors, as well as an agent in promoting mental and physical health and wellbeing.

Our social support not only affects our happiness and mental health, it also helps determine whether we'll die younger or older. In the study 'Social Relationships and Mortality Risk', no matter what cause of death the researchers looked at they found 'a 50 per cent increased likelihood of survival for participants with stronger social relationships'. They suggest the influence of social relationships on our risk of death is comparable to well-established risk factors for mortality such as smoking and alcohol consumption and that it exceeds that of other risk factors such as physical inactivity and obesity. Therefore, 'medical care could recommend if not outright promote enhanced social connections ... Individuals do not exist in isolation; social factors influence individuals' health through cognitive, affective and behavioural pathways.'

This shouldn't surprise us. Decades ago high death rates were observed among infants in orphanages, and even when researchers took into account other possible explanations, such as pre-existing health conditions, it was the lack of human contact that predicted their mortality: 'The medical profession was stunned to learn that infants would die without social interaction. This single finding, so simplistic in hindsight, was responsible for changes in practice and policy that markedly decreased mortality rates in custodial care settings. Contemporary medicine could similarly benefit from acknowledging the data: Social relationships influence the health outcomes of adults.'[4]

To give you an idea of how profound the influence of social support is, consider that even our genes are subject to 'social regulation', seemingly affected by our sense of social isolation or support. Genes within the small white blood cells of the immune system undergo global changes in people who feel high levels of social isolation.[5]

And social interaction with our acquaintances needn't always be pleasant: the Chinese University of Hong Kong studied the 'Benefits of negative social exchanges for emotional closeness' and found that insulting your friends may have an upside both for you and the person on the receiving end. Although, as they said, 'Negative exchanges in social relationships have traditionally been studied as having negative consequences' their research revealed that 'more negative exchanges were associated with a more positive change in closeness over a two-year period'.[6]

(Anti-) Social Networking

While debate continues over whether 'social media' help or hinder people, the way you use them is now a growing medical issue. Engaging in 'social comparisons' online is not good for your body image, according to the study 'Maladaptive Facebook usage predicts increases in body dissatisfaction and bulimic symptoms'. Writing in the *Journal of Affective Disorders*, the authors believe their results suggest that reducing 'maladaptive Facebook usage may be a fruitful target for interventions aimed at reducing body dissatisfaction and symptoms of eating pathology'. Social media enable us to make a large number of virtual social and physical comparisons and despite the term 'social media', the effect can turn out to be antisocial.[7]

A large team of scientists from the USA and Belgium published their study 'Facebook Use Predicts Declines in Subjective Well-Being in Young Adults' in the journal of the Public Library of Science. The study examined how Facebook use influences two central aspects of our wellbeing: how we feel moment to moment and how satisfied we are with our lives. They reported that Facebook use predicts negative shifts on both of these variables over time. 'The more people used Facebook at one time point, the worse they felt the next time ... the more they used Facebook over two-weeks, the more their life satisfaction levels declined over time.'

Their conclusions regarding higher levels of Facebook use are pretty damning, while those regarding the benefits of face-to-face interaction are positively glowing: 'The human need for social connection is well established, as are the benefits that people derive from such connection. On the surface, Facebook provides an invaluable resource for fulfilling such needs by allowing people to instantly connect. Rather than enhancing well-being, as frequent interactions with supportive "offline" [face-to-face] social networks powerfully do, the current findings demonstrate that interacting with Facebook may predict the opposite result for young adults – it may undermine it.' In fact, according to the study, 'direct social network inter-actions led people to feel *better* over time. This suggests that Facebook use may constitute a unique form of social network interaction that predicts impoverished well-being.'[8]

To be clear, mentioning the above studies is most certainly not an attempt to pin the blame for body dissatisfaction on Facebook. It is meant to draw attention to the way our direct interaction with one another has declined and how it has been displaced or replaced by something which may not provide the same benefits, leaving us more vulnerable to body dissatisfaction.

Displacement

The overuse of social media is now associated with other problems. Chapter 3, 'A Source of Thinspiration', described how the myriad idealised images transmitted through electronic media may contribute directly to body dissatisfaction. However, an equally important question is: what under-recognised things which could work against body dissatisfaction are being *displaced* by the time we spend with electronic media?

Several years ago I published a paper on how the increasing use of electronic media has coincided with a dramatic fall in eye-to-eye contact and face-to-face social interaction. The paper includes a graph that charts, in hours per day, the amount of time we have spent socially interacting face to face over the past twenty years. In the same graph, a second line charts the amount of time spent using electronic media. It is quite a sobering vision to see the two lines crossing around the year 2000, when virtual life took over from the real thing in terms of how we spend our time. And this crossover has, in my view, had the most profound implications for the way we view ourselves and feel truly supported and connected to others – or not.[9]

The overwhelming change in the way we interact is brought into sharp relief again and again when I find myself in foreign cultures in which few or no electronic media are available. The most notable difference is the amount of time that people spend looking at one another – children at their parents, for example – eye to eye. People also converse a lot more face to face. The tiny village of Anna Rais in central Borneo is well known for its beautiful natural surroundings and the uniqueness of its villagers' – the Bidayuhs' – way of life. They live in communal longhouses, raised off the ground on stilts, and each family can sit in the large front veranda area and talk either between themselves or with one another. After visiting the house of severed heads containing metal basketfuls of skulls from the victims of the village's headhunters of yesteryear, I opted for a civilised chat with the village elders. And even there, on the other side of the world, I found the same pattern emerging as screens arrived in the village. With the best of intentions the government wanted the tribe to be connected to the same information available to those in more urban areas, yet one of the most pronounced immediate effects was to displace the time the families spent talking and looking at one another and interacting with other families on the verandas.

The dramatic increase in, say, Internet use, along with the corresponding drop in face-to-face contact, has led researchers at Stanford University to develop a 'displacement' theory of Internet use: 'In short, no matter how time online is measured and no matter which type of social activity is considered, time spent on the Internet reduces time spent in face-to-face relationships ... an hour on the Internet reduces face-to-face time with family by close to twenty-four minutes.'[10]

And there was a similar reduction in face-to-face time with friends too.

While many bloggers, net-loving columnists and commentators may claim these are selective studies giving a distorted account of how high amounts of social networking may not be best for our sense of wellbeing, medical societies and government departments do not agree and have advised against spending too much spare time online. Excessive screen time is strongly linked with lower measures of mental wellbeing among children and young people in, for example, the American Academy of Pediatrics' use of the term 'Facebook Depression' mentioned previously (see p. 60).

A growing number of governments now advocate limiting all

discretionary (non-work/school) screen time. The Department of Health's Public Health England, for instance, has recommended 'rationing children's non-homework screen time ... The evidence suggests a "dose–response" relationship, where each additional hour of viewing increases children's likelihood of experiencing socio-emotional problems and the risk of lower self-esteem.' And they mention that 'specific types of internet activity (social networking sites, multi-player online games) have been associated with lower levels of wellbeing among children.'[11] The US Department of Health in their 'recommended limits for screen time' advises that children from the age of two up to eighteen should 'view television, videos or play video games ... use a computer or play computer games outside of school (for non-school work) for no more than two hours a day'.[12] Like many substances or other forms of exposure, from foods to alcohol to time spent in direct sunlight, screen time is now considered a form of consumption. And excessive consumption may have consequences.

Our face-to-face time has no lobby group; there's nothing to manufacture or sell, which explains why corporations aren't promoting the medicinal benefits that we as human beings can provide for one another *without* any of their products or services. The point is that by investing an increasingly large proportion of our lives in the cyber world, we are inadvertently neglecting a profound source of emotional strength and resilience that could help prevent and reduce body dissatisfaction. So until proven otherwise, when it comes to social interaction, keep it real.

Who Cares?

While it's good for your mental and physical health to be on the receiving end of social support, there's now convincing evidence

151

that it may be even better to give than to receive. Giving to or helping others works directly against an attentional bias towards self-focusing – a key problem in body dissatisfaction – because you are, without necessarily being conscious of it, focusing on others. And beyond this, knowing you are making a difference to someone else's life may unconsciously raise your sense of self-worth, which again is good for lowering body dissatisfaction.

Researchers at Harvard Business School recently published a study in the *International Journal of Happiness and Development* – incongruous though that may seem. They carried out three studies of charitable donations, or more precisely 'pro-social spending', and found that spending money on others or giving money to charity leads to the greatest happiness boost when giving fosters social connection. The overarching conclusion was that donors feel happiest if they give to a charity via a friend, relative or social connection, rather than simply making an anonymous donation to a worthy cause.[13]

Other studies are finding that more altruistic attitudes, volunteering and informal helping 'make unique contributions to the maintenance of life satisfaction, positive affect and other wellbeing indicators'.[14]

The University of Michigan's Institute for Social Research looked at 400 older married couples and found that those who provided social support to their spouses or practical support such as transport and childcare to relatives and friends, reduced their chances of dying by between 40 and 60 per cent in a five-year period. The authors thought the effects of these altruistic acts were surprisingly powerful and that there could be an as yet unidentified evolutionary advantage gained from helping others.[15]

How giving and helping others translates into feeling better and being healthier is slowly being worked out. In a paper published in the *American Journal of Public Health* researchers found that helping other people reduces your likelihood of dying earlier by buffering the effects of stress which contributes to an earlier death.[16] Big-time mainstream medical publications such as the Journal of the American Medical Association's *Pediatrics* are now reporting that 'adolescents who volunteer to help others also benefit themselves, suggesting a novel way to improve health'. Why? Because regular volunteering appears to reduce substances in the bloodstream which increase the risk of cardiovascular disease such as heart attacks and stroke. In people who regularly volunteered to help others, blood levels of interleukin 6 (which regulates immune system responses) and cholesterol were lower, as was their body mass index.[17] At the other end of the age spectrum, in people over fifty-seven to eighty-five, blood tests showed that those who helped others had lower levels of C-reactive protein, another compound strongly linked to cardiovascular disease.[18]

Hallelujah

As a devout agnostic, I've noticed that a growing number of people seem to feel that organised religion is uncool, even oppressive. This, in turn, has given rise to what I see as closet Christians: those believers who practise their faith rather discreetly. A secular society is increasingly promoted as a more modern, enlightened one. However, as the importance of religion has been declining in industrialised countries, scientists are finding noteworthy links between spirituality and better health. Those who were brought up with some sort of faith, but have become lapsed worshippers, or sinners, may want to consider dusting off their Bibles and getting back into practice – or perhaps booking a confession to repent.

Despite differences in rituals and beliefs among the world's major religions, spirituality is correlated with having better mental health, regardless of faith, according to University of Missouri researchers. They believe it may help by reducing self-centeredness and developing a sense of belonging to a larger whole. They examined the health of Buddhists, Muslims, Jews, Catholics and Protestants. Across all five faiths, a greater degree of spirituality was related to better mental health, specifically lower levels of neuroticism and greater extraversion. One of the researchers said, 'With increased spirituality people reduce their sense of self and feel a greater sense of oneness and connectedness with the rest of the universe.' He added that the benefits of a more spiritual personality may go beyond an individual's mental health in that the selflessness that comes with spirituality enhances characteristics that are important for fostering a world based on the virtues of peace and co-operation.

Researchers have also found that religious and spiritual support improve health outcomes for both men and women who face chronic health conditions and disabilities, including spinal-cord injury, brain injury, stroke and cancer. Support involved a variety of different things, ranging from spiritual interventions, such as religious counselling and forgiveness practices, to assistance from pastors and hospital chaplains.[19]

Neuroscientists at the University of Toronto asked religious people and non-believers to carry out a well-known cognitive task. Compared to non-believers, the religious participants – or even those who simply believe in the existence of God – showed considerably less activity in the anterior cingulate cortex (ACC), a part of the brain which can act like an alarm bell that rings when an individual has just made a mistake or experiences uncertainty. In other words, they were much less anxious and felt less stressed on making errors. These findings suggest that it is the calming effect of religious belief on its devotees that makes them less likely to feel worried about slipping up or facing the unknown.[20]

In a further more specific study they found that when people are primed to think about religion and God and then asked to carry out a very difficult task, their brains respond differently and in a way that lets them take setbacks in their stride and react with less distress to anxiety-provoking mistakes. Interestingly, atheists reacted differently; when they were unconsciously primed with God-related ideas, their brains' ACC increased its activity. The researchers suggest that for religious people, thinking about God may provide a way of ordering the world and explaining apparently random events, thus reducing feelings of distress. In contrast, for atheists, thoughts of God may contradict the meaning systems they embrace and thus cause them more distress. Atheists shouldn't despair, though. The lead investigator Professor Michael Inzlicht believes that these effects may occur with any meaning system that provides structure and enables people to make sense of their world. Inzlicht suggests that perhaps atheists would do better if they were primed to think about their own beliefs. 'We think this can help us understand some of the really interesting findings about people who are religious. Although not unequivocal, there is some evidence that religious people live longer and they tend to be happier and healthier.'

And there may be additional benefits to believing. In a series of four experiments published in *Psychological Science* investigators found that 'religion replenishes self-control' and improves our ability to make decisions. When the scientists made it difficult for people to succeed at tasks that required greater self-control, they found that implicit reminders of religious concepts 'refueled people's ability to exercise self-control ... religion had a unique influence on self-control.'[21]

But it isn't a question of praying for salvation from hating your cankles. It's a matter of looking closer to home for greater inner strength and fortification against life's adversities, including the pressures on body image. Many people may take their quiescent religious background for granted, like a lot of the other resources and fixtures of support around us that have faded into the background. Shifting our focus and attentional bias from ourselves, combined with the benefit of resilience that religion may bring means that in the face of body dissatisfaction we need to value it.

Common Experience: Same Time, Same Place

Communing with one another is also important. It sounds modern to speak in grander terms about our sense of place in the world, and I often hear people regurgitate phrases such as 'we live in a global world'. Yet although we are technologically global, this does not reduce our need to also feel a sense of connection to the people and places that are physically around us. It is, at times, still as important as ever to experience the same things at the same time in the same place. To put it technically, we need more 'co-presence' in 'real time'.

Societies I've seen where people share more common experiences appear healthier; and individuals who share more common experiences are happier and healthier too.

While technology and media offer the sense of global interconnection, it's important to ask whether this is actually a true sense of mutuality or a virtual one? Having simultaneous but separate experiences is not the same as sharing a common one. Even misery deserves real company.

Take, for example, our greatest single discretionary waking activity – recreational screen media from TV to the Internet. Investing so much of our time looking away from home erodes the consideration we have for our own geographically real communities by deceiving us into feeling that we are in some abstract way part of a larger world community – connected within a more important scheme of things. Furthermore, this new sense of omnipresence – events and images of people, values and lifestyles with which we often have little connection and even less control over – can add to an ever-growing sense of impotence and inadequacy.

It is a sense of real shared experience and connection closer to home that buffers us against the effects of the fast changes our culture is undergoing. Ballet dancers say that the way they prevent dizziness and nausea while pirouetting is to keep sight of one spot. This constant reference point enables them to cope with the rapidly spinning and changing landscape before their eyes. And the same is true of us in a more general sense.

Reinforcing various forms of shared or common experience and preserving our sense of place provides a feeling of control over our lives. The need to maintain and strengthen our sources of common experience is, in effect, a social medicine. And in trying to bolster our resilience to adversity, including pressures and negative feelings about our bodies, more common experience provides a firmer grounding to fight back from.

Pets

Those who are averse to communing with one another or with God may prefer (wo)man's best friend for social support. It is assumed by many that pets are good for you: lowering blood pressure, extending your life and making you happier than if you were petless. (Whether this applies to being the proud owner of home-reared tarantulas is unclear.)

Upon publication of 'Pet Ownership and Cardiovascular

Risk: A Scientific Statement from the American Heart Association', the lead scientist stated, 'Pet ownership, particularly dog ownership, is probably associated with a decreased risk of heart disease.' The studies aren't definitive and do not necessarily prove that owning a pet directly causes a reduction in heart disease risk, although research has found that owning pets may be linked with lower blood pressure and cholesterol levels, and a lower incidence of obesity and that pets can have a positive effect on the body's reactions to stress.[22] Female friends of mine have informed me of further benefits: 'If they become difficult or aggressive, you can make an appointment to have them "fixed".'

In a study in the journal *Society and Animals*, university students who chose to live with at least one dog, one cat or a combination of the two were less likely to report feeling lonely and depressed – something they directly attributed to their pet. Avoiding loneliness was the top reason given by both students and adults whether married or single.[23] A study published by the American Psychological Society reported that dogs increased their owners' feelings of belonging, self-esteem and meaningful existence. The authors wrote that there is 'considerable evidence that pets benefit the lives of their owners, both psychologically and physically, by serving as an important source of social support'.[24]

Considering body dissatisfaction, one thing that a pet will force you to do is focus on *them* instead of just yourself: shifting your attention and locus of control. And of course, you benefit from caring for 'someone' else too. Your pet depends on you, and looking after another creature, providing for its needs, can help give you a sense of your own value and importance. If you have a dog, it needs to be walked and, as has been discussed (see Chapter 8, 'Running Away from Body Dissatisfaction'), that extra activity is good for your physical and mental health, including body dissatisfaction. An animal's natural routine – say, waking you in the morning, demanding food or walks – also provides a structure, which can, in turn, be quietly reassuring in its constancy.

There is also a degree of social interaction and support: companionship. If you have a pet, you're never alone. And they can indirectly lead you to have more social contact. You might chat with other people while walking your dog at the park or waiting at the vet. Pets are a consummate pretext to talk and other pet owners love to discuss their animals. A dog can be better than a dating agency.

Ultimately, pets can provide unconditional and uncomplicated love – you don't have to worry about hurting your pet's feelings or getting advice you don't want. Of course, there are always people who take this too literally: twenty-nine-year-old Emily Mabou of Aburi, Ghana reportedly married her eighteen-month-old dog in a ceremony attended by a traditional priest and local, curious villagers. This was because, she said, 'For so long, I've been praying for a life partner who will have all the qualities of my dad. My dad was kind, faithful and loyal to my mum, and he never let her down. I've been in relationships with so many men ... and they are all the same ... skirt-chasers and cheaters. My dog is kind and loyal to me and he treats me with so much respect.'

It isn't always consensual, however. In February 2006 a Sudanese man named Charles Tombe was forced to take a neighbour's goat as his 'wife', after he was caught *in flagrante delicto* with the animal. The goat's owner, Mr Alifi, said he surprised the libidinous man with his goat and took him to a council of elders who ordered Mr Tombe, to pay a dowry of 15,000 Sudanese dinars to Mr Alifi who said, 'We have given him the goat, and as far as we know they are still together.'[25]

Scientists have yet to work out whether such bonding and social support improves body image in goats.

159

Ten

Altered Images

In addition to bolstering our resilience to the influences that create or heighten negative thoughts about our bodies, psychologists have confronted head on the thoughts lying behind body dissatisfaction, by teaching women, literally, to alter them, i.e. 'Nothing's changed, so I've decided to change my mind.'

Forget about the ids, egos and superegos, along with the Oedipal complex and 'Why did you hate your mother?' of Freudian psychoanalysis. Given the intensive conditioning most Western women have undergone, resulting in what some call the 'internalisation of the thin ideal', there is now evidence that some counter-conditioning of your thoughts can also be achieved through therapeutic approaches such as cognitive-behavioural techniques or dissonance-based interventions. These newer therapies do less introspection through the rear-view mirror and involve, for example, a structured series of verbal, written and behavioural exercises requiring you to critique the thin-ideal standard of female beauty that has been burned into your psyche. In the case of dissonance-based interventions researchers claim the intervention effects are very robust, producing 'significantly larger reductions in thin ideal internalization, body dissatisfaction, self-reported dieting, negative affect [negative emotions]'.

While this may sound like off-the-shelf pop therapy, it's not. There is growing evidence that cognitive behavioural and other therapeutic approaches may actually change the way our brains function and maybe even the way they're wired. Studies looking at the 'neurobiological effects of psychotherapy' through brain imaging carried out before and after a course of therapy, are concluding that 'a psychotherapeutic approach, such as CBT [cognitive behavioural therapy], has the potential to modify the dysfunctional neural circuitry associated with anxiety disorders. They further indicate that the changes made at the mind level, within a psychotherapeutic context, are able to functionally "rewire" the brain.'[1]

Psychological therapies are now also being closely studied for their measurable physiological effects. For example, anxiety and stress in cancer patients seem to cause the immune system to allow inflammation through changes in the behaviour of genes in the white blood cells. However, a fascinating study by the University of Miami found that cognitive-behavioural stress management seemed to reverse this process in breast cancer patients.[2] Furthermore, the 2013 annual conference of the European Society of Cardiology heard that psychological interventions halve deaths and cardiovascular events in heart-disease patients.[3]

The point in describing these studies is to show that what may seem lightweight talking and thinking may actually bring about more powerful changes than we might otherwise have thought.

Dissonance-based Interventions

We generally crave consistency and prefer to act according to our beliefs, and so become troubled when we find ourselves doing things we don't believe in. The idea behind 'dissonance theory' is to harness our desire for consistency. We're asked to behave in ways similar to people with healthier behaviour and ideas about body weight. In a structured group situation, for instance, by being asked to write letters to hypothetical younger girls, warning them about the risks of idealising slimness, it is hoped we too may change our feelings about the need to be slimmer and therefore about being unattractive. We may also be asked to make lists of the top ten things girls can do to resist pursuing the 'thin ideal' with the aim of changing our own feelings about embracing the values which make us feel worse about our own bodies. Most of the activities take place in a group setting, in line with research that suggests we're more likely to adopt ideas which we've proclaimed publicly. Add to this the distinct possibility that misery may very well love company.

The main proponents of dissonance-based interventions believe that this approach for eating disorders tends to be significantly more effective than others. One of the studies followed people over several years and found they still benefitted three years after the group sessions. Dissonance-based prevention programmes are also thought to have saved lives by preventing fatal eating disorders.[4]

The researchers also note that the same approach may be effective in reducing negative attitudes (e.g. racism) and in promoting healthier behaviours in relation to drinking, smoking, safe sex and even conserving water. So although altering attitudes in order to alter behaviour may seem the obvious way round, evidence suggests that altering the behaviour first and allowing attitudes to follow suit might be more effective: I am, therefore I think. A new review of this general approach concluded that there was generally positive evidence for the effectiveness of dissonance-based interventions.[5]

Cognitive Behavioural Therapy

Cognitive behavioural therapy (CBT) also attempts to reduce your problem by changing the way you think and behave. It encourages you to examine how your actions can affect how you think and feel. By looking at your situation and either talking about it or writing it down in a structured way, it's thought you can change how you think and what you do, thereby enabling you to feel better and more able to manage.

Unlike therapies such as psychoanalysis, CBT addresses your current problems, rather than dwelling on your past and seeks practical ways to improve your state of mind on a daily basis. It attempts to help you make sense of problems by breaking them down into smaller parts with the idea that your thoughts, feelings, physical sensations and behaviour are interconnected, often locking you into a negative self-reinforcing pattern. CBT tries to directly interrupt these negative cycles by identifying and separating the factors that are making you feel less than comfortable, so that they may become more manageable and thus improve the way you feel.

CBT is adapted by different therapists, but with respect to dealing with body dissatisfaction the process may follow a variation of the following pattern:

• First, you carry out a self-assessment of how your negative body image may have developed – your case history.

- Second, you learn to keep a diary about events that surround body dissatisfaction.
- Third, there is relaxation training and/or 'mindfulness' to accept current body-image experiences and to accept and then 'neutralise' negative body-image emotions – 'private body talk'.

You are then taught to identify and adjust errors in your body-image judgment, along with self-defeating, avoidant or evasive and compulsive body-image behaviours; you learn different strategies to reduce these negative behaviours; and, ultimately, you review the new cognitive and behaviour skills and learn how to implement them in difficult interpersonal events that provoke negative body image.

CBT usually involves a session with a therapist once a week or once every two weeks. Overall, the number of sessions you need will depend on your individual problems and objectives, but therapy usually lasts from six weeks to six months – a relatively short period compared with other talking therapies. (This is one reason the private American health insurance companies took to it like a duck to water.) However, to benefit from CBT, you need to apply yourself to the process and invest time, thought and effort into working through the various stages. A therapist can help and advise you, but they need your full commitment.

There are also self-help manuals involving a systematic programme of therapy which you can work through. For many people a CBT self-help manual will be good enough to improve their body-image problems, so they can lead better lives without enlisting the services of a therapist. Many women are reluctant to get professional help because they feel they haven't made a serious enough effort to deal with it by themselves. Others feel body dissatisfaction is too 'trivial' and would be embarrassed to look for help. Still others are simply ashamed of their bodies to the extent that they cannot bring themselves to tell a therapist. Besides, good professional help is not always easy to come by and the process can often seem too daunting. A self-help manual is very helpful in these cases, if only to break the ice on body dissatisfaction.[6]

It's important to reiterate that there are times when body dissatisfaction may be one aspect of a deeper, more complex problem such as anorexia, bulimia, binge-eating disorder or body dysmorphic disorder. In such cases, a programme based entirely on self-help is going to be less helpful than treatment managed by a suitable therapist.[7] Further information is provided in the Resources section (see p. 247).

Eleven

In Our Own Image

'Girls don't simply decide to hate their bodies, we teach them to.'

There is, undoubtedly, a strong element of social transmission in our children's body dissatisfaction: from society, culture and peer groups. But they also get free hand-me-downs from us.

Although children's body image has been addressed through separate books on adult and on child body issues, this is a false distinction. How we adults fare and feel about our own bodies is often linked to how our children fare and feel about theirs: parents who hate their bodies are more likely to produce children who hate their bodies too. By treating these issues separately, we've compromised our ability to confront them and break the cycle of an epidemic now considered literally contagious.

Parental Transmission

Girls are *very* interested in body fat and body shape. That's nothing new. What is new is the extent to which they're interested, the age at which the interest becomes pronounced and what they're willing to do to their bodies in order to achieve what they want. And boys too are following suit with a desire for muscle and a leaner, more low-fat, defined look (see Chapter 6, 'Manorexia').

So how do we pass our body dissatisfaction on to our children? And how can we stop its transmission and replace it with self-esteem-enhancing alternatives?

Our daughters and sons are affected by most of the same things that affect us. The main differences are that they are still developing their own identity and sense of self, are far less able to distinguish between realistic and unrealistic judgments and expectations and are far more susceptible to media images. However, beyond these factors is our central role in influencing our daughters' body image. And although scientific attention has begun to focus in particular on the inadvertent effects that mothers have on their daughters' body image, fathers do play a part too:

> Father to mother: 'I'm surprised you could fit into that
>   swimsuit this year.'
> Mother to father: 'Right! You're sleeping on the sofa!'

Not good. As an initial guide to masculine values and preferences, fathers are priming their daughters with a template to make value judgments about themselves and others. Daughters can pick up fundamental biases via this type of interaction between their two main role models.

A study of over 5000 ten- to eleven-year-olds by the US government's Centers for Disease Control and Prevention found that in addition to the role of peers in cultivating or preventing body dissatisfaction, parents mattered big time. They found that 'mother nurturance' was related positively to a child's 'physical self-worth' for girls, and father nurturance was related positively to physical self-worth for boys. In turn, greater physical self-worth, for both boys and girls was related to greater body satisfaction.[1] Moving up in age, another study on body dissatisfaction in eleven- to sixteen-year-olds again found peer influence was important, but that 'parental encouragement to control weight and shape was a strong predictor of weight concerns in boys and girls alike'.[2]

A mother's feelings about her own body and her own dieting can affect not only her child's body image, but their BMI as well. A study in the journal *Appetite* looked at how a mother's self-image and dieting may actually lead to a weight change in her two-year-old child and found 'maternal dietary restraint directly predicting change in child BMIz [a mathematical variant of BMI] over the year'. They went on to report: 'Mothers' BMI and body dissatisfaction may contribute indirectly to weight change in their young children. Interventions targeting maternal body dissatisfaction and informing about effective feeding strategies may help prevent increases in child BMIz.'[3]

As body dissatisfaction and, to some extent, anorexia are increasingly seen to be socially transmitted, mothers are being advised not to talk about dieting in front of their children or to complain about parts of their body they don't like. Placing a lot of emphasis on and making comments about weight and body shape, combined with idealised images of slim celebs, is bad for our children's self-esteem. So although you may not feel great about your body, by remaining seemingly neutral or positive about the way you look, you'll be helping your child to develop their own body confidence.

The good news is that studies are finding that effective communication between you and your child works in favour of their body satisfaction. It may not surprise you to hear that your general relationship with your child – girl or boy – is related to their body image. (As mentioned early on, children can also use eating and over-exercising to express conflict or unhappiness, including that involving parents.) For example, research by the Division of Adolescent Medicine, Boston Children's Hospital found that 'a more positive mother–adolescent relationship predicted lower body shame and higher body esteem in adolescents, suggesting that the quality of the relationship with the mother may be a protective factor for adolescents' body image'. They advise health professionals that for interventions aimed at improving children's body image, the quality of the mother–adolescent relationship is a clear point of entry. Therapists should, they say, work with adolescents and their mothers on the quality of their relationship in order to impact positively on adolescents' body image.[4] While this is good news it's also a responsibility that weighs heavily (so to speak).

Beyond its influence on body dissatisfaction, parenting can influence a child's self-esteem, which overlaps with body satisfaction. So as parents we can be reassured – or worried – to hear that an Australian study of seven- to eleven-year-olds found that 'parental responsiveness showed a positive association with child self-esteem ... A responsive parenting style may assist in promoting child self-esteem.'[5]

Giving our children our regular undivided attention will enable them to get things off their chest that could otherwise be potentially expressed through feelings about their body or through food and dieting.

Solutions

The following are a range of factors that may help protect our children from the pressures on their body image.

Mastering mastery

As with adults, getting our children to involve themselves in pursuits that engage them, provide them with a sense of control, competence and accomplishment – 'mastery experiences' – may indirectly cultivate greater body satisfaction, partly because they're spreading their risk and putting the eggs of their self-esteem in more than one basket. And by investing themselves in things that give them a sense of satisfaction and competence, they're not only shifting their attention away from feelings about their bodies, but also gaining a more general sense of influence over their lives, making them more resilient in the face of cultural and peer pressures.

Looking outward

Returning to the basic theme of shifting of attention and self-focusing, children need to alter their focus and emotional resources away from bodies and appearance. If they're engaged elsewhere, they simply have less emotional and intellectual room and time for feeling or thinking about bodies. It's the body-image version of 'the devil finds work for idle hands' principle.

Enculturating our children to help others and to think and feel for others will rob them of the time and resources to think about themselves and their bodies. Thinking more about others will also have widespread benefits for our entire society and can make an historical difference to how our times will be remembered.

But as it stands, psychometric measures of the 'dark side' of self-regard – or narcissism – have risen steadily in the young since the early 1980s. A US national study of 16,475 college students concluded that today's young are more narcissistic and self-centred than their predecessors. Two-thirds of students have above-average scores of 30 per cent more than a quarter of a century ago.[6] New technology contributes further. What with MySpace, YouTube, selfy, Facebook and Twitter, it's no exaggeration to suggest that It's All About Me. Because, according to recent research, it is. A meta-analysis of seventy-two studies on empathy over thirty years involving almost 14,000 university students offers little flattery for the young: 'College kids today are about 40 per cent lower in empathy than their counterparts of twenty or thirty years ago.'[7] By confronting the cult of individualism and the self in the next generation we may not only be making a more pleasant future for ourselves, we'll be creating a more pleasant future for them. Thinking of and caring about others has to be encouraged and cultivated by parents and, if it is, it may help our children's body image.

As was discussed earlier for adults (see Chapter 9, 'Well Connected'), helping other people addresses a key problem in body dissatisfaction of an attentional bias towards self-focusing, because by helping others children will be focusing outward. And feeling that they may be making a difference to someone else's life may help with self-esteem which may, in turn, help body esteem. There are many ways in which children can do this, either on a casual, ad-hoc personal basis within the extended family or neighbourhood or through more organised means – Scouts, Brownies or other community or school schemes and activities involving volunteering and informal helping.[8]

Puberty

Discussions with your child about their body-image concerns should be linked with discussions of puberty because the two are inextricably tied. And while you're at it, you can mention how genes and hormones influence size, shape and body fat distribution too. Whether you want to hit them with, 'And so, what I'm trying to say, darling, is that in the end, we all finish up looking like our mothers,' is entirely up to you.

The main difference that we can see between prepubescent girl, pubescent girl versus an adult woman is the accumulation of body fat on her hips, thighs and bottom as she reaches full adulthood. These are the secondary sexual characteristics that develop with puberty which widens the pelvis and increases the amount of body fat in hips, thighs, buttocks and breasts.

Telling children that big changes in body shape – i.e. body-fat distribution – are good and necessary and that everyone develops at different times and rates, can be very reassuring. Most girls will begin puberty between eight and fourteen years of age, with the average age being eleven, and with most girls reaching full sexual maturity within four years.

It's also worth explaining to them some of the facts about female shape from Chapter 2, 'Know Your Wiggle Room', on, for example, the necessity of having more gluteofemoral fat and why it is actually considered attractive to boys. This is the very opposite of the messages our culture is forcing on them, and will give them a very different perspective . . . and a compelling one at that.

In the same way that girls may not be aware of the extent to which their stage of puberty, genes and hormones may influence their size, shape and body-fat distribution, boys too are ignorant of the fact that their rate of becoming more muscular is partly genetic and also limited by their age. And there is even greater variation than with girls. Boys tend to develop later than girls, and the process usually takes longer: most boys begin puberty at nine to fourteen years of age, with most reaching maturity within six years. Most importantly, testosterone is vital for muscle development and some boys are naturally endowed with higher levels than others, and will therefore have more muscle and an easier time building it. You may not want to give them the bad news that testosterone levels peak around the age of thirty, long after their sexual-performance peak of age eighteen.

In response to your child lamenting, 'Why can't I look like her/him?' you can remind them of the genetic and puberty stage differences between people of the same age. And you can point to how boys of exactly the same age differ in musculature, size and height and how you as an adult differ in body shape and size from your friends and even your sister(s), if applicable.

Role modelling

You are generally the most influential role model in your child's life, and although it is not easy to feel self-assured about your body all the time, as we've already seen, by appearing to be at least neutral about it, you will help prevent your daughter from picking up less than constructive messages. So save the complaints about the parts of your body you hate until you're out of earshot, thereby shielding her from what could be referred to undiplomatically as psychic contamination.

In addition to keeping your self-opinions low-profile it's a good idea to do the same to your bathroom scales, diet sheets/books and anything else overtly relevant to you not liking your body and wanting to change it. Using scales judiciously for medical reasons is, of course, another matter because the object appears different to that of physical-appearance goals. But too much mirror-gazing, especially with a frown on your face, is not good (and it's not good for you either): out of sight out of mind.

Encourage the straightforward enjoyment of food without thinking about its meaning so much: less cognitive eating, along with moderate physical activity, as opposed to fit-and-toned calorie-defying exercise.

It's more important than ever to help our children develop

173

values other than consumerism. Children often absorb our values ambiently without us having to make them explicit. Your teenager may, on the surface, appear to despise your values, but they are still highly likely to become infected with them. (Haven't you ever found yourself thinking, 'Oh my God, I sounded exactly like my mother just then'?) Share some of your values with your children and create opportunities for them to immerse themselves in as many of them as possible – such as enjoying nature, reading, the arts, sports, music, cultivating friendships, volunteering or other activities. It's a matter of engaging your children in life outside their body awareness. Unless there's a problem, you needn't sit your child down and drill them about their 'body image'; instead, you'd be better off asking them their opinions on what's was going on in the news, what they're learning in school and nurturing their existing interests, resulting in them being too involved in other aspects of their life to remember to be interested in how much they weigh.

And let's not forget also that the vast majority of our children will themselves become parents, so it's high time we broke the cycle of pregnancy or post-pregnancy being considered a visual tragedy for women (see Chapter 5, 'Baby Dissatisfaction').

Ageist comments

We have to face the facts: as a result of sustained low fertility and increasing life expectancy the population of most developed countries is ageing. While this book has confined itself to body image in terms of size and shape, rising right along with body dissatisfaction is its chronological counterpart: our culture's 'gerontophobia' – fear of growing old, or a hatred or fear of the elderly. If we want to be respected as we age and not thought of as hideous, and if we want to spare our children an accentuated unease about their appearance as *they* age, we have to stop and think about our culture's sheer revulsion at ageing and our growing disrespect for the elderly.

And charity begins at home. Commenting disparagingly about your own or others' ageing looks is passing on a value system, which will make us and our children unhappy. If your child sees a television programme or magazine criticising someone for their wrinkles or other signs of ageing, pick them up on it.

More male input

Men, meaning in this case fathers and even grandfathers, have a very different and much kinder take on female body fat, sex appeal, eating and weight loss. Mothers and other women need to harness this different perspective and ensure it's put to good use.

Most fathers are relatively oblivious to how very sensitive their daughters may be about their bodies, yet would not be amused to think that their little girls are being bullied by a culture of slimness. What they do about it in their own clumsy way is another matter, as many fathers aren't sure how to – or if they should – approach their daughters. They're typically more comfortable coaching their sons in football and talking about the latest sports scores. It may be that many fathers don't understand themselves as being that important to their daughter's body image and general self-esteem. However, a good relationship between father and daughter can have many benefits for a daughter, such as being more self-reliant, self-confident and successful and less likely to develop body-image problems and eating disorders.[9] Fathers often relate to their daughters by doing things together that they both enjoy. In interviews with adult women that I read, I often hear how influential such father–daughter experiences were and how they shaped their interests and goals.

Of course, fathers are also husbands and partners, and so

how (or *if*) they say things about the body/appearance of their daughters' primary role model – you – it can have an indirect impact on their daughter's body-image concerns, as mentioned earlier. On the other hand, a father saying, 'You look wonderful,' to either mother or daughter is rarely a bad move.

And a note about brothers: boys and men in general are more prone to practical jokes and the joys of overt taunting. I am more guilty than most. In fact, I've been planning to patent my invention, which is only a pipe dream at the moment: the spousal-taunting stick. My device would enable the lazy husband to physically annoy his wife without having to leave the comfort of his lazy-boy reclining chair. The advert would run:

'Make the timeless art of annoying your wife easier than ever – but from a safe distance and with a built-in Taser in case it all goes wrong. Available in standard or deluxe with gold relief handle. *Includes free life insurance.'

We men prod around a female's psyche and find what she reacts to and then press that button in order to elicit the predictable response. When a boy discovers that telling his sister she has corn-on-the-cob calves or the plumpest of posteriors produces shrieks of pain, discomfort and rage, this is likely to make him very happy because he now knows how to effortlessly annoy his sister. Have a word with him about this though, as he is unlikely to realise the profound longer-term implications of teasing his sister about her body.

It is also worth sitting your daughter down and explaining this proclivity that some boys have for provoking in a seemingly insensitive and cruel way. I see it all the time: while teenage boys may adore the pear shape, they will nevertheless taunt girls about their hips and thighs purely to get a reaction without understanding the significance of what they've said.

Body movement for body image

Getting your child involved in physical activity now – whether through organised sports or otherwise – can set them up with good habits and better health for life.

And it may also improve their grades as well as helping to prevent or reduce body dissatisfaction: considering the obesity problem among children in most industrialised countries, new research indicates that physical activity may be the key to reducing kids' waist size while increasing their brain size.

A study published in *Brain Research* has found an association between physical fitness and the brain anatomy in nine- and ten-year-old children. Those who were more physically fit tended to have a bigger hippocampus – about 12 per cent larger, relative to total brain size – and perform better on a test of memory than their less fit peers. (The hippocampus is important in learning and memory, and a bigger hippocampus is associated with better performance on spatial reasoning and cognitive tasks.)[10]

The American Heart Association reported that children who are aerobically fit 'over time score the highest mean on all the academic sub-tests'. And the brain-versus-brawn issue takes another twist in a study of 1.2 million Swedish male teenagers published in the *Proceedings of the National Academy of Sciences,* which found that teenagers who are fit have a higher IQ and are more likely to go on to university. But it is only cardiovascular fitness not muscle strength that plays a role in the IQ test results; the researchers think that cardiovascular fitness ensures that the brain gets plenty of oxygen.

The study also found that teenagers who improve their physical fitness between the ages of fifteen and eighteen increase their cognitive performance when measured at age eighteen: 'This being the case, physical education is a subject that has an important place in schools, and is an absolute must if we want to do well in maths and other theoretical subjects.'[11]

Physical activity is thought to help a child's cognitive processing by increasing blood and oxygen flow to the brain. This raises levels of norepinephrine and endorphins to decrease stress and improve mood, and increases growth factors that help create new nerve cells and support the connections between brain cell synapses that are at the basis of learning.

Studies of brain function at the Medical College of Georgia on seven- to eleven-year-olds have found a direct, positive relationship between their level of physical activity and that of frontal-lobe brain activity (blood flow) – an important area for intellectual executive function. Furthermore, these brain changes correspond directly with positive changes in pupils' cognitive test scores, assessing their decision-making processes and maths achievement.

The message should be very clear: children must spend at least an hour a day doing some form of moderate to vigorous physical activity, vigorous being much better than moderate.

As mentioned in Chapter 8, 'Running Away from Body Dissatisfaction', physical activity can also provide all of us, children included, with 'mastery experiences' (see p. 138).

A study entitled 'The Effects of Aerobic Exercise on Psychosocial Functioning of Adolescents Who Are Overweight or Obese' found that even without losing any body fat, the children's body image improved in relation to the physical exercise alone. They also reported improved 'perceived scholastic competence and social competence'.[12]

Physical activity may also be a route to cultivating healthy eating habits in our children. Research by the Université de Sherbrooke in Quebec compared children who engage in about an hour of physical activity daily with those who are sedentary and found the physically active children were generally more likely to eat fruit, vegetables and whole-grain foods and to have breakfast. They recommend that 'there should be particular actions targeting students in the last half of primary school, aimed at developing individual accountability and autonomy with respect to healthy eating and physical activity'.[13]

Media literacy cure?

Media literacy consultants have been quick to offer schools help in developing pupils' skills to manage media influences through encouraging them to think more critically about media messages and images that promote unrealistic body shapes – 'helping children to understand what they see'. But should they be seeing so much of this in the first place? And can we explain the effects away after the fact? No and no.

There are profound limits as to how far we can redress through rational explanation what is a cumulative *subconscious* emotional effect. The average person sees 1500 adverts per day on top of the many more slender idealised images they see in non-adverts.[14] Exposing photos as being airbrushed cannot negate the effects of seeing a high number of unrealistic images for many hours a day. After all, if it doesn't protect adult women from body dissatisfaction why expect it to protect children? Media people want our children to learn to 'consume media critically', but what they don't want is for our children to simply consume less media full stop. Because, as stated earlier, 'the money's where the eyeballs are'.

There's no escaping the need for children's self-evaluation to involve more non-virtual points of comparison – i.e. real people. While 'social media' sites promise greater human connection, engaging in 'social comparisons' online is not good for body image.[15] It is, therefore, important to encourage children to spend more time off-line in the real world and less in the virtual one so they are able to compare themselves within a healthy arena. Yet another good reason to reduce screen time (see pp. 59–60).

Of course, in a general sense it's important to ensure that from a young age our children understand the inconsistencies between what is real and what has been altered in media images, and to help them see the impact the media can have on the way they feel about their appearance. And it's also important for all of us to encourage our children to question and challenge Western society's (literally) narrow 'beauty ideal'.

Reducing our children's exposure to a high volume of idealised images from media is vital. However, it is equally vital to ensure that the sheer amount of time they spend looking at media doesn't displace the time they could spend doing and experiencing things that may be good for them and which may bolster their resilience to pressures on their body image. A few final general themes appear in many advisories for parents which are summarised here:

- Help our children to be more accepting and less judgmental about other people's body shapes and sizes. Bitching in agreement with catty magazines or judges on the *X-Factor* about appearance is easy to do, but our children then learn from two sets of role models – the media and their own parents – that being nasty about bodies is good.
- Challenge the visual conformity dished up by the media by helping our children to see that there are many forms of beauty aside from those they routinely see on TV and in magazines, etc. There are plenty of examples in Chapter 4, 'What Men Want', and unless you explain some of this alternative information to your child, the media – their main waking activity – certainly isn't going to.
- When we talk about people in general we should try and place more emphasis on their personal attributes as opposed

to the way they look – their character, achievements, talents, abilities and outlook on life, for example. Ask your children to think about some of the people they know and love. What is it that they love about them?

- Help siphon off your child's worries about their body by simply listening: a problem shared is often a problem halved, just because it's been aired. Offering reassurance to concerns about body image from your vantage point of age and experience does help to prevent these negative themes from becoming embedded in your child's thinking.

- If you do become worried about your child's body concerns, eating or body weight, don't think for a minute that you're the only one or a hysterical mother. Liaise with their school over pressure and signs of body-image problems that warrant attention. Intervene if your daughter's friend is becoming too thin or if her peer group is involved in a dieting competition. Talk to other parents, if possible.

Parental Support

Unconditional love, that unique phenomenon that mothers in particular give out to their children, is a powerful antidote to the insecurity-rousing messages our kids are bathed in. Let them know how we feel about them – provided it's good news – and let's try to place more value on their efforts and achievements. Encouraging children to recognise and pursue their own talents, skills and other strengths helps inoculate against body dissatisfaction by shifting their centre of gravity to other confidence-boosting areas of their lives.

Although the relationship between social support and body dissatisfaction is complicated and not exactly clear, within families there is some evidence that social support can be an important factor in preventing/reducing body dissatisfaction.[16] One practical suggestion is simply to eat together as a family more frequently. The American Medical Association's main paediatrics journal published a five-year study of 2516 adolescents by epidemiologists and consultants in adolescent medicine which found that eating together as a family is so important it should now be considered a health issue: 'Healthcare professionals have an important role to play in reinforcing the benefits of family meals ... Schools and community organisations should also be encouraged to make it easier for families to have shared mealtimes on a regular basis.' The study found, for example, that adolescent girls who frequently eat meals with their families are less likely to use diet pills, laxatives or other extreme measures to control their weight five years later, 'even after adjusting for sociodemographic characteristics, body mass index, family connectedness, parental encouragement to diet and extreme weight control behaviours'.[17] This has been followed by a study in the official journal of the American Academy of Pediatrics, encouraging doctors to consider advising patients 'about the benefits of sharing three or more family mealtimes per week; these include a reduction in the odds for overweight (12 per cent), eating unhealthy foods (20 per cent) and disordered eating (35 per cent) and an increase in the odds for eating healthy foods (24 per cent).[18]

Ultimately, however, preventing body dissatisfaction in our children is often less a case of actively doing and saying positive things and more a case of doing and saying fewer negative things. The concept of 'celebrating our bodies' is an adult one; children's bodies shouldn't be objectified. If anything, they should be thought about less, talked about less and merely taken for granted.

Twelve

Downsizing

Calories
(noun)
Tiny creatures that live in your closet and sew your
clothes together a little bit tighter every night.

If body dissatisfaction is more about 'feeing fat', irrespective of
how fat you may or may not actually be, then you are likely to
have dieted and may well try again in future. But as was made
clear in Chapter 2, 'Know Your Wiggle Room', it's absolutely
imperative that you first gauge your BMI, waist-to-hip ratio
(WHR) and possibly your percentage of body fat to determine
if you need to reduce your BMI. You can use the tools in
Chapter 2 and in the Appendix (see p. 208) to get a clear
answer. Alternatively, your GP's surgery can do it for you.

   If you do genuinely need to lose weight, remember any diet
can enable you to do so, but keeping it off is invariably a spectacular failure, which is why diet companies continue to stay in
business for decades. The key to successful weight loss – i.e.
loss of excessive body fat, especially intra-abdominal fat – is in

making changes to your eating and physical activity habits that you can keep up for the rest of your life.

Many people may nod their heads and agree with this last statement intellectually, but emotionally they cling to a belief in a Next New Thing which will 'deliver' the slimmer figure they want: a Messiah Diet. While research continues to *refine* our understanding of the main factors that cause us to gain and lose excess body fat, there is no Next New Thing. Many of the answers are openly available now and they're free – something we apparently find hard to believe. We harbour a masochism which assumes we must spend pounds to shed pounds and that there are weight-loss 'tips' and 'dieting secrets' which will deliver us from plumpness.

As a case in point, there seems to be a general belief that the recent wave of low-carbohydrate, high-fat diets are in some way 'new' or 'revolutionary'. They are not. In 1863 William Banting, a formerly obese English undertaker, became the first person to popularise a weight-loss diet based on limiting intake of refined carbohydrates. In his pamphlet *Letter on Corpulence, Addressed to the Public* he outlined the details of a particular low-carbohydrate diet that had led to his own dramatic weight loss. The diet was called 'Banting' and was such a success that the question 'Do you bant?' referring initially to his method, was eventually used in the context of dieting in general.[1] Jump forward 150 years and we have Banting's offspring in the form of the paleolithic diet or 'caveman diet': eat like a caveman and you'll look like Fred Flintstone's wife Wilma. And then, of course, there's the Atkins diet. So ... the Next New Thing?

A Losing Battle

In the quest to *remain* slimmer, diets don't work. Diets as we commonly know them – sudden temporary reductions in calories to lose weight – are a 'major medical event'. The British Dietetic Association, the professional association and trade union for dietitians – whose job it is to consider weight loss and what we eat – makes it clear: 'It is important not to "diet". Diets are often extreme, strict and nutritionally unbalanced and dictate what you should and shouldn't eat resulting in you not sticking to them for very long ... Remember there is no quick fix. People who successfully lose weight and keep it off stay realistic and develop techniques to make their new lifestyle and activity habits an enjoyable way of life.'[2]

And just to ensure that any lingering remnants of a diet dream are completely shattered it's worth repeating here that dieting is increasingly being found to cause significant metabolic, neuroendocrine and epigenetic changes, in some cases leading to disease (see p. 40).

Regaining weight is often attributed to a drop in 'motivation' or our inability to stick to the diet and exercise, but biology also plays an important role. After losing weight, the rate at which we burn calories (energy expenditure) slows down, reflecting our slower metabolism. Lower energy expenditure adds to the difficulty of maintaining our new weight and helps explain why people tend to regain the weight they lost.

Body fat is an active part of your endocrine (hormone) system, providing feedback for hunger and diet to the brain. So what you do to your body fat – for example, dieting or starving it – can change the way it behaves and how it grows. Furthermore, it's thought that some of us may inherit more brown fat (see p. 30) and/or our brown fat is more easily activated to burn our white body fat, which may keep us slimmer with little effort.[3]

It's beyond the scope of this book to provide a comprehensive guide on how to lose weight. Nowadays, many health departments have interactive websites and GPs' surgeries often have links with dietitians who can advise you, and there are many credible (and free) sources of information listed in the Resources section of this book (see p. 247). It is, however, important to dispel the myriad wrong assumptions about weight loss as a necessary reality check and as a block to resorting to dieting to deal with body dissatisfaction. To be clear, there's nothing wrong with losing body fat if you genuinely need to for straight-forward health benefits. And there are, on occasion, medical reasons to lose weight through a prescribed diet by a doctor or under the care of a hospital. But dieting is not the answer to body dissatisfaction if you do not need to lose body fat. And as was made clear early on, body dissatisfaction often has little to do with how fat or slender you actually are, and much more to do with how you *feel* about your body's appearance. So don't link weight loss with greater happiness – it doesn't work that way.

Given the high level of body dissatisfaction prevalent in our society and the hijacking and confusion over fat loss and dieting, it makes sense to separate the health reasons for losing body fat from dealing with how we feel about our body shape and size.

Fat Facts

Why do so many people get fat? On the surface the reason seems obvious. The World Health Organization states: 'The fundamental cause of obesity and overweight is an energy imbalance between calories consumed and calories expended' – we either eat too much or are too sedentary or both. The remedy you'd think is also obvious: eat less, exercise more. But as you'll see, the solution is more complex and nuanced than a simple input/output model of fatness.

It's important to get a feel for the basic mechanisms involved in preventing obesity and reducing body fat in a healthy, enduring way in order for you to later decide what specific courses of action you can take to lead a healthier and reduced-fat life – if that's what's medically required.

There's no avoiding having to learn some of the key principles of nutrition or else you'll be eating out of the palm of the diet industry's hand for the rest of your life. You'll also be at the mercy of the food industry whose first priority is to fatten up their bank balance, not slim down your waistline. But if you do get a feel for the fundamentals of nutrition, you'll be permanently equipped to make better decisions about what you eat intuitively, without having to count calories or eat so consciously. You'll just have a sense of what to put on your plate, whether it's in your kitchen or at a restaurant buffet. Further sources of practical information about the basic food facts can also be found in the Resources section (see p. 247). In the meantime, here's some food for thought:

All calories are not equal

We may have to now re-evaluate the fattening potential of the foods we eat as new research challenges the idea that a calorie is a calorie.

There are many types of carbohydrates (carbs) – or starchy foods – but they all behave differently in your body. This is because they are digested at different rates, which has an effect on your blood-glucose (blood-sugar) levels. A scale called the glycaemic index (GI) is used to rank how quickly different foods make your blood-glucose levels rise after eating them.

There is some research to suggest that slow, steady rises and falls in glucose may help control appetite. And a study published in the *Journal of the American Medical Association* has found that diets which reduce the surge in blood sugar after a meal – either low-GI or very low-carbohydrate may be preferable to a low-fat diet for those trying to achieve lasting weight loss. Furthermore, the study finds that the low-glycaemic-index diet had similar metabolic benefits to the very low-carb diet, but without some of the negative effects of the latter.[4] 'From a metabolic perspective our study suggests that all calories are not alike,' said one of the researchers, Professor David Ludwig, at Harvard Medical School. 'The quality of the calories going in is going to affect the number of calories going out. The best diet from a metabolic perspective was the low-carbohydrate diet, but there were downsides ... The metabolic benefits of this diet may be undermined by more inflammation and higher cortisol, both of which can increase [heart disease and stroke] risk over time,' Ludwig said.[5]

Though a low-fat diet is traditionally recommended by the US Government and Heart Association, it caused the greatest decrease in energy expenditure, an unhealthy pattern in blood fats and insulin resistance (whereby cells in the body are unable to use insulin effectively, potentially leading to diabetes). 'In addition to the benefits noted in this study, we believe that low-glycemic-index diets are easier to stick to on a day-to-day basis, compared to low-carb and low-fat diets, which many people find limiting,' says lead author Professor Cara Ebbeling. 'Unlike low-fat and very-low carbohydrate diets, a low-glycemic-index diet doesn't eliminate entire classes of food, likely making it easier to follow and more sustainable.'

It should be pointed out that there is not, as yet, a consensus on exactly how useful the GI will ultimately prove to be. It is not a magic bullet for weight loss – the amount you eat is also important and not all low-GI foods are necessarily good for you. In general, however, filling lower-GI foods such as beans, peas, lentils, porridge, muesli and most fruit and vegetables are good choices and can help you to manage your weight and keep to an overall healthy eating plan.

Carbohydrate food	Lower GI Choice
Bread	Multigrain, granary, rye, seeded bread, wholegrain pita bread, chapatti, oat bread
Potatoes	New potatoes in their skins, sweet potato, yam
Pasta	All pasta if cooked al dente, noodles
Rice	Basmati rice, long-grain or brown rice
Other grains	Bulgur wheat, barley, couscous, quinoa
Breakfast cereals	Porridge, muesli, most oat and bran-based cereals

Alcohol

Another aspect of our lifestyle that can directly or indirectly contribute to weight gain is alcohol. Among adults who drink, alcohol accounts for nearly 10 per cent of their calorie intake. Yet most of us have no idea how many calories are in our drinks. Gram for gram, alcohol has almost twice as many calories as pure sugar and almost as many as pure melted pig's fat. It is also an appetite stimulant and can lead to overeating at mealtimes, late at night and even the next day. What's more, alcohol impairs your 'impulse control' while you're tipsy, which could lead to unbridled piggery.[6]

Exercise

There is no consensus as yet on how effective exercise is in weight loss. It does seem that what we eat is the more important of the two. It's more than a matter of simply burning calories; exercise also affects the hormones that control appetite – in particular ghrelin, which stimulates hunger. So while exercise may indeed burn calories, some believe that ultimately, it makes us prone to eat more later.

However, a 2012 study from the University of Wyoming examined women who either ran or walked and, on alternate days, sat quietly for an hour. In each case they were then directed to a room with a buffet. The researchers found that when the women ran, their ghrelin levels spiked, which should have meant they would pig out at the buffet. Not so. In fact, they ate several hundred fewer calories than they burned. The walkers overate, consuming more calories at the buffet than they had burned, and the same was true after sitting. Why? Because the runners produced additional appetite-suppressing hormones only recently discovered telling their bodies they'd eaten enough and could stop. These additional hormones in effect 'muted' the message from the hunger hormone ghrelin.[7] So it seems the type of exercise we do also has a part to play in how much we eat.

Another study looked at the longer-term effects of exercise on appetite with some interesting findings. Scientists at the Department of Cancer Research and Molecular Medicine, Norwegian University of Science and Technology, looked at the effects of 'chronic exercise', i.e. moderate exercise – the equivalent of brisk jogging. They found that after twelve weeks, overweight people who were formerly sedentary began recognising, without consciously knowing it, that they should not overeat. The scientists even secretly doctored their milkshakes to see how their appetites would react when they were then given free reign at a buffet, as well as how much they ate later in the day, but it seemed their appetite-control mechanism had improved over the three months to the point where it could judge the amount of calories consumed earlier and adjust for that afterward. This type of 'chronic exercise' seems to hone our body's satiety mechanisms. But the message is to think not in immediate calorie-burning terms, but in the long term: when it comes to weight loss and its maintenance, longevity counts. You need to stick with it in order to fine-tune appetite control.[8]

Resistance exercise

We may not be able to override a genetic predisposition to gain weight easily, but building muscle may fortify our bodies to a degree and delay the point at which our figures start to widen with age. However, muscle mass begins to diminish as you reach menopause, so eventually, your body will probably start nudging its way outward. If you do some resistance training – for example, light weights or even some heavier gardening – and stay physically active into your fifties, you'll put on less weight.

As with how we eat, which shouldn't involve short-term diets, physical activity too must be an ambient, integral, long-term part of the way we lead our lives and not a special 'procedure' to lose weight.

Spot reduction?

Fitness magazines and advertisements want us to believe we can lose body fat in the specific areas that trouble us – so by doing exercise which selectively targets certain body parts, we can supposedly bring about 'localised fat loss'. Scientific studies suggest otherwise. The fat that's broken down to be used as fuel during prolonged exercise can come from anywhere in your body, not just the part that is being exercised the most. You're more likely to melt down your love handles by regular jogging than by doing crunches and sit-ups every day, simply because cardiovascular exercise is a much more efficient calorie-burner. Doing 150 crunches a day can certainly strengthen your abdominal muscles, but it probably won't make them any more visible and you can end up hiding your six-pack under a bushel.

Chapter 2, 'Know Your Wiggle Room', went to great lengths to help explain our width, pointing out the different types of body fat and the differences between the various key areas in which it's located. And with good reason: because fat disappears from some parts far more easily than from others. As exercise physiologists Sharon Plowman and Denise L. Smith have reported, the ability to reshape your glutefemoral fat pattern (your pear shape) is extremely limited because it is driven and supported by your hormones. This shouldn't be depressing, but liberating; it means not that you're doing something wrong or bad, but rather that your pear has security guards which are pretty intolerant to any embezzlement of its stored assets. Fat cells in our abdominal region (apple shape) are, however, more 'unstable' and more easily bribed to get lost.[9]

Monthly menu?

Most women seem to suspect that their appetite or cravings are influenced by their menstrual cycle and they're probably right. Scientists at Oxford University's Nuffield Department of Obstetrics and Gynaecology did find that women ate more at certain times of the month: 'Intakes of carbohydrates, protein and fat were significantly higher in the pre-menstrual phase than in the menstrual phase.'[10] And the Human Appetite Research Unit, Institute of Psychological Sciences, University of Leeds found that sugars and alcohol were both consumed in greater amounts in the pre-menstrual phase in women with pre-menstrual syndrome.[11] Understanding this could be significant in people trying to lose weight, as regular phases of eating more calorie-dense foods add up. We mustn't undervalue the potential influence of the female menstrual cycle on eating.

The TV Diet?

According to a study by the private healthcare company Bupa, 'The average Brit walks only ten minutes a day during the working week,' and one in five admits to not leaving their desk all day except to 'use the bathroom or grab a drink'. Furthermore, the younger generation (eighteen- to twenty-four-year-olds) is apparently the least active with a massive 25 per cent of them 'only walking when it's necessary and needing someone to walk with to get them motivated enough to start'. In looking for explanations most parents said, 'Technology could be to blame.' The direct implications for body fat are too obvious. Little wonder then that Bupa has launched its Ground Miles campaign to get people moving on foot.[12]

In addition to the effects of slender images on the psyche and the fact that too much screen time may displace or negatively affect our social support systems, technology – be it YouTube, DVDs, computer games or television – is of significant interest to doctors in trying to prevent obesity, diabetes and cardiovascular disease. For example, a team of doctors observed changes in the arteries of thirty-two-year-olds over a four-year period and found that by the time they reached thirty-six the 'time spent watching television is associated with arterial stiffness'. This effect was quite independent of and couldn't be explained by other possible influences, such as a lack of exercise or 'other lifestyle risk factors ... Given the independent associations of time spent watching television ... our study suggests that not only promotion of physical activity, *but also* discouragement of sedentary behaviours should be targeted in younger adults to prevent arterial stiffening.'[13]

I published a medical paper entitled 'Time for a view on screen time' in the British Medical Journal's *Archives of Disease in Childhood* which goes into the issue in far greater detail.[14] Here are some of the most relevant points:

- In addition to simply being sedentary, our recreational screen time (the discretionary time we spend on our screens outside of work) is now considered a separate *independent* factor in gaining body fat, above and beyond just being lazy and sedentary. To be precise, even though you're sitting on your ass, screen viewing is *not* the same as sedentary behaviour.
- The link between screen time and body fat appears even stronger in young children. A British study assessing 'fat mass' found a 'dose–response relationship': 'Each extra hour of watching TV was associated with an extra 1kg of body fat ... Preschool children who watch more TV are fatter and are less active ... the relation between TV viewing and fatness is not mediated by physical activity.'[15]
- Increased TV viewing has been consistently shown to be linked to increased body mass index (BMI) in both children and adults, independent of the amount of physical activity they get. The association appears stronger in young children and may be long-lasting. Community health researchers at University of Montreal recently published a study with the self-explanatory title 'Early childhood television viewing predicts explosive leg strength and waist circumference by middle childhood'.[16]
- Studies of eating behaviour in direct response to screen viewing suggest that looking at a screen can act as a distraction away from critical satiation food cues toward non-food cues (screen), thereby inhibiting the development of feeling full when presented with more food and, therefore, increasing calorie intake while we are viewing. Eating a meal while watching screens is also thought to disrupt the brain's ability to encode and memorise what we eat. So when we see food hours

later our brain may be less able to reconcile what we ate before with what we could eat now, and this may increase our food consumption hours after our screen viewing stops. In this study, women were more likely to raid the cookie jar.

And all these effects are taking place at a time in our history when 68 per cent of dinners in the UK are eaten while people are watching television.[17]

Cutting screen time to fight obesity is now a serious medical initiative. In addition to the screen-time guidelines mentioned earlier in this book (see p. 150), the EU ToyBox study group of doctors has called for 'limitation of leisure screen time to less than one hour per day' in its 'evidence-based recommendations for the development of obesity prevention programs' for young children.[18] If we, as adults, want to be a healthy weight and shape, we should take their advice too. Because screen time is *not* the same as other forms of sedentary behaviour and has additional independent effects which may produce additional body fat.

This gives a whole new meaning to the term 'wide-screen TV'.

Big friendships

And while we're at it, why not blame our friends too? It seems that they too are a part of the definition of that 'obesogenic environment' we're exposed to. Earlier on I mentioned the links between our friends' body image and weight and our own body satisfaction – or lack of it (see p. 10). Well, there's also a link between our friends' obesity and our own. Scientists have proposed the 'social-norm hypothesis', whereby 'social affiliation fosters shared norms or ideals (e.g. about the acceptability of being overweight), which then lead to similarity in body mass index (BMI) through the actions of these ideals on diet and physical activity'.[19]

A study by researchers at Harvard Medical School published in the *New England Journal of Medicine*, using longitudinal data from the thirty-two-year Framingham Heart Study, found that being fat appears to be socially contagious, especially via our mutual friendships, over time: 'Obesity appears to spread through social ties. These findings have implications for clinical and public health interventions.'[20]

A further study published in the *American Journal of Public Health* confirmed this conclusion and found that if you have heavier friends, family members, and colleagues, it is more likely that you will be heavier too: the stronger the relationship between two people, the stronger the link between their weights. The explanation, they suspect, is a case of monkey see, monkey do: you change your eating habits to mirror those of your friends without necessarily thinking or talking about an ideal body weight. One of the researchers gave an everyday example of this mechanism: you're at a restaurant with friends and the waiter brings over the puddings menu. Everyone else decides not to order anything, so you pass too, even though you were dying for a piece of Death by Chocolate Cake.[21]

The health advice isn't to ditch all friends and disown brothers, sisters and parents for the sake of your hips and thighs, but rather, simply to be aware of the possible influence of others on you. And perhaps your own influence on others next time you say, 'Oh, go on – have another tub of Ben & Jerry's'.

Big mistakes?

It should be clear that our weight and weight loss are influenced by many things above and beyond our self-discipline and willpower. The Academy of Medical Royal Colleges representing all of the main Royal Colleges of medicine and surgery is quite convinced it isn't simply 'our fault' that we're overweight. They're certain it's the environment we're exposed to that makes it inevitable and that drastic legislation is needed urgently to curb its fattening effects on us. Their national report 'The Medical Profession's Prescription for the Nation's Obesity Crisis', which focuses on 'changing the "obesogenic" environment' and 'making the healthy choice the easy choice' sounds rock'n'roll radical. The first words of the report are hardly political comfy-speak: 'The UK is the "fat man" of Europe.' And given that there's no money in it for these doctors if we lose weight, or even if we gain it, we should believe their version of why we have an obesity problem. This applies to other countries too, where doctors' views are overshadowed by the big money of food-and-drink-industry lobby groups and by politicians. Despite the seemingly neo-liberal thought that nutrition and health are all about 'personal choice', controlling your appetite and weight is *not* that simple.

The Academy of Medical Royal Colleges' 220,000 doctors are, for example, demanding a 20 per cent increase in the cost of sugary drinks, fewer fast-food outlets near schools and a ban on television advertisements for foods that are high in salt, sugar and saturated fat before the 9 p.m. watershed, as the current measures to minimise our children's exposure to them have not worked.[22]

Coming full circle back to body dissatisfaction, research now finds that improving our body image *first*, may actually enhance the effectiveness of weight-loss programmes based on healthy eating and physical activity. The authors go on to say: 'From this we believe that learning to relate to your body in healthier ways is an important aspect of maintaining weight loss and should be addressed in every weight-control programme.'[23]

Thirteen

War and Peace

To think that we stand at a point in our social history where it is now abnormal for a woman to be satisfied with her body shape should strike all of us as both astonishing and perverse. And to think that scientists have had to develop the term 'normative discontent' to describe this state of affairs should be chilling. To consider that this term is increasingly accurate in describing the way three- to six-year-old girls feel about their bodies should be intolerable, making us fiercely angry and protective.

And so we stand at a defining moment, surveying a future where fewer and fewer girls will have known a time when it wasn't absolutely normal to be unhappy with your body. Such a prospect must, surely, galvanise us to change their future – and ours too.

To 'fight back' on so many fronts – personal, educational, cultural and political – may seem overwhelming and unfeasible. But picking our battles wisely can reap an accumulation of modest yet appreciable victories. The media, our culture and our own deeply entrenched feelings, values and judgments about our bodies are not going to surrender to sense overnight. After all, we're fighting fundamental norms and multi-billion-dollar industries that continue to perpetuate and profit from what they have helped to cause.

It's therefore vital that we focus initially on trying to influence those areas of our lives that we can, and accept those we can't. So instead of notions of banishing body dissatisfaction from our lives and learning to love our bodies happily ever after, we should aim simply to lead less troubled, healthier and more fulfilling lives: to merely feel more comfortable with our size and shape. Recapping, this means the following:

- A reality check on what is possible is a good factual point from which to start confronting body dissatisfaction. The vital first step is to use legitimate yardsticks on body size and shape in making judgments (see Chapter 1, 'Size Matters') in order to narrow the gap between what we want and believe is possible versus what is realistic and healthy.
- Mustering up greater resilience to the ubiquitous pressures from both within and without can subtly cause a sea change in emphasis and perspective in your feelings about the way you look. The measures outlined earlier in Chapters 8–12 may seem unremarkable, but they are a prerequisite for good mental and physical wellbeing, whether you experience body dissatisfaction or not.
- Shifting our attention, focus and emotional resources from our bodies and appearance will help to chase the ghost of body image away or at the very least keep it from the front door. Redistributing our emotional and intellectual resources to a more realistic balance by involving ourselves in other areas of life that engage us, will provide us with a sense of control, competence and accomplishment, and work strongly in favour of us feeling better about the way we look.

- In the age of the self, it is important to look outward to others, whether through caring and helping (or through religion, God forbid). Yes, there are personal gains to be had here, but it is also of benefit to other people and to our society. And again, shifting attention away from body concerns and, for that matter, away from yourself, gives you the time and distance that are unavailable to you in the day-to-day world of body dissatisfaction.

- Children in particular need to spend less of their spare time in the virtual world, filled as it is with idealised images, and more of it in the real world where their comparisons involve real people. Reducing consumption of – or exposure to – a source of discontent is an obvious need. As a powerful, long-overdue measure, this will provide many benefits and prevent problems for people of all ages.

- All of us need to reclaim eating from being a considered 'act' and return it to being something we simply do and enjoy. Cognitive eating, as aided and abetted by TV, magazines and books, should be identified and driven away from our dinner tables. The same goes for appearance-based 'exercise' and terms such as 'fit and toned', now a byword for something very different. There should be no negotiation with the hijackers of these formerly innocent concepts.

- Wrenching the yardstick for making judgments about our bodies away from the food, diet and fashion industries must be accompanied by new ground rules, making it absolutely clear that there is a terrible conflict of interest at play and that these sources are *not* to be trusted when discussing dress size, body-fat distribution, body size and weight, what is attractive or healthy and, most of all, what is in our best interests. These interest groups are marketeers, *not* arbiters of what's best for our health and wellbeing.

- With the diet industry emphasisng *our own* role in

establishing our level of body fat, we must remind ourselves that it is not merely a question of self-discipline and personal choice, and that what we are surrounded by and tempted with has a direct effect on our body size, weight and shape. Given the constraints of our genetic disposition and the obesogenic environment in which we live, there is only so much we can do.

- Public education to prevent or, at the very least, counteract the damaging cultural messages to which children in particular are increasingly exposed is vital. Some researchers are speaking in terms of 'universal interventions targeting entire schools and communities'.[1]

- Enlightening our children by explaining the way idealised media images work must not be seen as an open-house invitation for media viewing under the educational guise of 'media literacy'. Rational explanation is in no way a substitute for protecting them from seeing the harmful images in the first place and will not simply negate the effects of doing so. There are profound limits as to how far we can inoculate our children through intellectual explanation against what is a cumulative *subconscious* emotional effect.

- There's also an important moral issue at stake in encouraging girls to understand what they see in the media as being artificial because the subtext is, 'It's *your* perception that's the underlying problem, little girl – it's not us, it's *you* that needs re-educating.' As the fashion and beauty industries increasingly attempt to airbrush their image through various 'social responsibility' initiatives, we must all bear this in mind. Don't let them get away with it; there is a conflict of interest.

- While schools have been trying to 'get down with the kids' by using hip celebrities (particularly slim, attractive ones) to 'make learning more relevant', a rethink of this school-endorsed reverence for the beautiful people is strongly advised – idealised images are, after all, still idealised images.

- As parents we are generally the most influential role models in our children's lives. This provides an opportunity for us to halt the transmission of body dissatisfaction from parent to child, by being more careful about what we say/do about our own bodies in front of our children. We can also try to ensure that our values about bodies and appearance work against those of the media that are freely available in our homes.

- The assumption that confronting body dissatisfaction is 'wimmin's business' has deprived us of a vast resource of heavy reinforcement, namely men – or, in other words, husbands, partners, fathers, grandfathers and brothers. Instead of being wrongly viewed as the cause of the current situation, they should be welcomed into the resistance movement, both within families and at a more political level.

- There are times when body dissatisfaction may be one aspect of a more deep-rooted body-image problem. We therefore need an improved general awareness of the need for proper therapeutic interventions, and our society requires greater resources in order to provide this. Dealing with body image or eating disorders early and effectively is a good example of 'an ounce of prevention is worth a pound of cure'.

Institutional Dissatisfaction

As with any drive to improve the health of the public, collective action is also required – and perhaps never more so than in reversing widespread body dissatisfaction. However, the latter continues to find institutional support, even at the level of our government. Such support may be inadvertent and unknowing, but we need more joined-up government involving the right departments with the right priorities to provide a more united front, enabling more cohesive action.

A good example is the British government's Body Confidence Campaign, run, not by the Department of Health, whose sole focus is the health and wellbeing of the nation, but by the Department for Culture, Media & Sport which describes itself as 'here to help make Britain the world's most creative and exciting place to live, visit and do business ... to give the UK a unique advantage in the global race for economic success'. They're joined by the Government Equalities Office 'responsible for equality strategy'. Both are 'advised' by the government's 'Advisory group' on body dissatisfaction – the Women's Business Council.

The widespread body dissatisfaction that so concerns the government should be tackled by the Department of Health, not by a media department, nor by an Equalities Office, nor by the Women's Business Council. Body dissatisfaction and its strong link with eating disorders with a high mortality risk is not merely an issue of 'media literacy and equality'.

In many countries governments have 'equality and diversity' legislation for employment and related areas of society. And many industries do the same. In Britain, the government even has 'Fairness for All' and a Human Rights Commission (EHRC) to get busy 'Building a Fairer Britain' by protecting, enforcing and promoting equality across nine 'protected' grounds – age, disability, gender, race, religion and belief, pregnancy and maternity, marriage and civil partnership, sexual orientation and gender reassignment.'[2]

And broadcasting organisations, you would have thought, should have to comply with 'equality and diversity' legislation both off screen and on.

Enter the Creative Diversity Network (CDN), representing the big-time UK television industry whose explicit aim is 'to promote, celebrate and share good practice around the diversity agenda ... to ensure that television continues to represent all parts of British society, both onscreen and within the industry.'[3] Their members all have diversity manifestos. For example, the British Academy of Film and Television Arts (BAFTA) has a website making their 'Diversity Pledge'.

The most fervent member of all is the BBC, the world's oldest national broadcasting organisation and its largest broadcaster by number of employees. Being a public service broadcaster, it gets its money from you.

The Beeb displays a voracious appetite for diversity. They have a Head of Diversity in their Diversity Centre, blogs from the Diversity Centre, the BBC Trust Equality & Diversity website and an ongoing BBC Equality Analysis. And there's a vision: the BBC's Diversity Strategy 2011–15, 'Showcasing the UK's complexity and diversity – on and off air'. All of this is accompanied by predictable corporate comfy-speak, for example, 'Diversity matters for all audiences and across all programme genres. Our youngest viewers take a matter-of-fact approach to difference, and it is important that we recognise and reflect this in our programmes.' This is accompanied by a photograph of a BBC Children's TV presenter with her right arm missing just below the elbow. But true to form, even the BBC's diverse version of disability was still clearly very slender.

Even the casting of a corpse in a forensic drama lying on a slab during an autopsy seems to favour the willowy dead-model look. Size 16s aren't wanted – dead or alive.

Interestingly, within all the politically correct diversi-babble, any mention of not discriminating against women with a normal body shape or size is conspicuous by its absence. The inclusivity rhetoric to 'portray life in the UK as it truly is' stops abruptly when body size is mentioned.

The BBC's Diversity Strategy embraces the law's Equality Act 2010 – the Public Sector Equality Duty, welcoming 'the responsibility on the BBC, as an organisation, to consider how it can advance equality of opportunity for people irrespective of their own characteristics ... requiring us to be transparent and open.'

However, there's a legal loophole allowing them to be excused from having to obey the law on equality and diversity: 'Exempted activities include, for example, commissioning, production, casting, editorial policy.' And so are 'casting' and 'production' decisions which invariably exclude female presenters, actresses and interviewees of a normal body size justified 'in order to protect the BBC's editorial independence'. Going back to the research I conducted into the body sizes and fat distribution of female children's BBC TV presenters which revealed that, at the time, not a single presenter approached an average body weight with normal fat distribution, it seems that any enthusiasm to 'embrace diversity', wears thin when it comes to embracing the ordinary woman.

However, this is by no means just a British problem. Women's consistent exclusion from television and film on the basis of body size and shape is something that is not open for discussion with broadcasting organisations in most countries. And I'm not talking about hiring clinically obese women; I'm merely referring to those who are, for example, a size 12, *well below* the average dress size 16. Although a token unrepresentative example of someone who is not a size 6 may be thrown out as evidence that there is no body discrimination in casting, a look at the vast majority of female presenters, expert interviewees, 'weather girls' and, of course, actresses – especially during prime time – convicts broadcasters beyond any reasonable doubt.

At the same time as the size 12s are being locked out of the TV studio, and despite legislation on ageism, there's the serious ongoing problem of deselecting women who, even if they are a size 6, have grey hair and/or wrinkles. This applies to all electronic media networks in most industrialised countries. So while a male news anchor and reporter may be fifty-five and the proud owner of a lovely pot belly, our daughters are increasingly learning from television, that the women who are most knowledgeable and capable in most fields – from meteorology, to news, to sport to economics – are young and slim. Yet, the reality is that most women who know an awful lot about something and have the most experience in a given area are likely not to be younger, but rather older (and therefore not as slim) because they've spent many years doing what they do.

The Royal College of Psychiatrists' 'Statement on the influence of the media on eating disorders' makes it absolutely clear 'there is a lack of reality-based imagery' in today's media, 'leading to lowered mood, body dissatisfaction and eating-disorder symptoms.'[4] So given that both the British Medical Association[5] and the Royal College of Psychiatrists have for some time called for a diverse range of media physiques and ages, it's surely time we *all* started to make trouble.

Print journalists and health professionals should begin to hound broadcasters and governments incessantly, demanding a clear explanation as to how the standard practice of excluding women of a size 14 has anything whatsoever to do with editorial independence, before going on to demand a closing up of legal loopholes that are barring women of a certain dress size (and age) from our screens. Perhaps to start the healing process, we should begin to name and shame the body-image bandits responsible: casting directors, producers, directors and even commissioning editors should be held publicly accountable for their discrimination.

We may also need to show a new-found enlightened intolerance toward body images deemed harmful, possibly with their active exclusion according to their degree of risk to young female viewers. This may seem an extraordinary form of social medicine, but the evidence suggests that 'a lack of reality-based imagery' in media is causing health problems in a very large number of women and young girls. And their rights must take precedence over those of the permarexic TV presenters' and broadcasters' fatuous claims for 'editorial independence'.

Slimness Is Next To Godliness?

Beyond the worldly issues discussed above, a question remains: is the pursuit of slenderness ultimately a reflection of our society's unmet spiritual needs, with body dissatisfaction masking deeper yearnings for a sense of purpose that religions used to provide?[6]

In my view, body dissatisfaction serves partly as a lightning rod for many contemporary anxieties we have and rapid changes we continue to face. However, I believe this functional role for body concerns has been augmented by its spiritual counterpart. And I strongly agree with theologians who suggest that the pursuit of a better body shape is for many, acting like a religion predicated upon the misguided belief that in order to be happy, healthy and attractive, you must be slim. A secular religion with its own set of beliefs, myths, rituals, images and moral codes that encourage followers to seek 'salvation' through weight loss: a belief system whereby our bodies are flawed and our appetites sinful.[7] Yet even as a devout agnostic, I'm not averse to heeding some advice on worshipping false gods directly from the Almighty's biography: 'Do not believe every spirit ... for many false prophets have gone out into the world' (John 4:1–6).

In the end, it is up to us as individuals to stop the major conflict over the way we feel about our own bodies. And although we may continue to have small, isolated skirmishes, a period of détente could eventually lead to a lasting peace. And so perhaps it's time for the negotiations to start.

Appendix

The following information may be used in conjunction with Chapter 2, 'Know Your Wiggle Room'.

Determining Your Frame Size

- Measure the thinnest area of your wrist using a tape measure.
- Write down the measurement.

For women, under 1.57m (5 feet 2in):

- a wrist circumference of under 14cm (5.5in) means you have a small frame
- a wrist circumference of between 14cm (5.5in) and 14.6cm (5.75in) means you have a medium frame
- a wrist circumference of over 14.6cm (5.75in) means you have a large frame.

For women between 1.57m (5 feet 2in) and 1.65m (5 feet 5in):

- a wrist circumference of under 15.24cm (6in) means you have a small frame

- a wrist circumference of between 15.24cm (6in) and 15.9cm (6.25in) means you have a medium frame
- a wrist circumference of over 15.9cm (6.25in) means you have a large frame.

For women taller than 1.65m (5 feet 5in):

- a wrist circumference of under 15.9cm (6.25in) means you have a small frame
- a wrist circumference of between 15.9cm (6.25in) and 16.5cm (6.5in) means you have a medium frame
- a wrist circumference of over 16.5cm (6.5in) means you have a large frame.

If you have a large frame, subtract 10 per cent from your BMI score (see below) before seeing which category it falls under. This means that the healthy BMI for a person with a large frame is roughly 23–25.

Body Mass Index (BMI)

The body mass index has been around since Belgian scientist and statistician Adolphe Quetelet invented it in the 1830s as a measure for human body shape. It is considered an accurate gauge for people aged twenty to sixty-five. You can find your BMI by locating your height and weight on the table below. Alternatively, you can do it online using the 'BMI healthy weight calculator' at www.nhs.uk, the 'Adult BMI Calculator' at the US Government's Center for Disease Control and Prevention (www.cdc.gov), 'Calculate your BMI' at the Australian Department of Health (www.health.gov.au) or the 'BMI calculator' at the Heart Foundation in New Zealand (www.heartfoundation.org.nz).

height (m)

weight (kg)	1.38	1.42	1.46	1.50	1.54	1.58	1.62	1.66	1.70	1.74	1.78	1.82	1.86	1.90	1.94	1.98	weight (st/lbs)
150	79	74	70	67	63	60	57	54	52	50	47	45	43	42	40	38	23s 8
148	78	73	69	66	62	59	56	54	51	49	47	45	43	41	39	38	23s 3
146	77	72	68	65	62	58	56	53	51	48	46	44	42	40	39	37	22s 13
144	76	71	68	64	61	58	55	52	50	48	45	43	42	40	38	37	22s 9
142	75	70	67	63	60	57	54	52	49	47	45	43	41	39	38	38	22s 4
140	74	69	66	62	59	56	53	51	48	46	44	42	40	39	37	36	22s
138	72	68	65	61	58	55	53	50	48	46	44	42	40	38	37	35	21s 10
136	71	67	64	60	57	54	52	49	47	45	43	41	39	38	36	35	21s 5
134	70	66	63	60	57	54	51	49	46	44	42	40	39	37	36	34	21s 1
132	69	65	62	59	56	53	50	48	46	44	42	40	38	37	35	34	20s 10
130	68	64	61	58	55	52	50	47	45	43	41	39	38	36	35	33	20s 6
128	67	63	60	57	54	51	49	46	44	42	40	39	37	35	34	33	20s 2
126	66	62	59	56	53	50	48	46	44	42	40	38	36	35	33	32	19s 12
124	65	61	58	55	52	50	47	45	43	41	39	37	36	34	33	32	19s 7
122	64	61	57	54	51	49	46	44	42	40	39	37	36	34	32	31	19s 3
120	63	60	56	53	51	48	46	44	42	40	38	36	35	33	32	31	18s 13
118	62	59	55	52	50	47	45	43	41	39	37	36	34	33	31	30	18s 8
116	61	58	54	52	49	46	44	42	40	38	37	35	34	32	31	30	18s 4
114	60	57	53	51	48	46	43	41	39	38	36	34	33	32	30	29	17s 13
112	59	56	53	50	47	45	43	41	39	37	35	34	32	31	30	29	17s 9
110	58	55	52	49	46	44	42	40	38	36	35	33	32	30	29	28	17s 5
108	57	54	51	48	46	43	41	39	37	36	34	33	31	30	29	28	17s
106	56	53	50	47	45	42	40	38	37	35	33	32	31	29	28	27	16s 10
104	55	52	49	46	44	42	40	38	36	34	33	31	30	29	28	27	16s 5
102	54	51	48	45	43	41	39	37	35	34	32	31	29	28	27	26	16s 1
100	53	50	47	44	42	40	38	36	35	33	32	30	29	28	27	26	15s 10
98	51	49	46	44	41	39	37	36	34	32	31	30	28	27	26	25	15s 6
96	50	48	45	43	40	38	37	35	33	32	30	29	28	27	26	24	15s 2
94	49	47	44	42	40	38	36	34	33	31	30	28	27	26	25	24	14s 11
92	48	46	43	41	39	37	35	33	32	30	29	28	27	25	24	23	14s 7
90	47	45	42	40	38	36	34	33	31	30	28	27	26	25	24	23	14s 2
88	46	44	41	39	37	35	34	32	30	29	28	27	25	24	23	22	13s 12
86	45	43	40	38	36	34	33	31	30	28	27	26	25	24	23	22	13s 8
84	44	42	39	37	35	34	32	30	29	28	27	25	24	23	22	21	13s 3
82	43	41	38	36	35	33	31	30	28	27	26	25	24	23	22	21	12s 13
80	42	40	38	36	34	32	30	29	28	26	25	24	23	22	21	20	12s 8
78	41	39	37	35	33	31	30	28	27	26	25	24	23	22	21	20	12s 4
76	40	38	36	34	32	30	29	28	26	25	24	23	22	21	20	19	12s
74	39	37	35	33	31	30	28	27	26	24	23	22	21	20	20	19	11s 9
72	38	36	34	32	30	29	27	26	25	24	23	22	21	20	19	18	11s 5
70	37	35	33	31	30	28	27	25	24	23	22	21	20	19	19	18	11s
68	36	34	32	30	29	27	26	25	24	22	21	21	20	19	18	17	10s 10
66	35	33	31	29	28	26	25	24	23	22	21	20	19	18	18	17	10s 6
64	34	32	30	28	27	26	24	23	22	21	20	19	18	18	17	16	10s 1
62	33	31	29	28	26	25	24	22	21	20	20	19	18	17	16	16	9s 11
60	32	30	28	27	25	24	23	22	21	20	19	18	17	17	16	15	9s 6
58	30	29	27	26	24	23	22	21	20	19	18	18	17	16	15	15	9s 2
56	29	28	26	25	24	22	21	20	19	18	18	17	16	16	15	14	8s 11
54	28	27	25	24	23	22	21	20	19	17	17	16	16	15	14	14	8s 7
52	27	26	24	23	22	21	20	19	18	17	16	16	15	14	14	13	8s 3
50	26	25	23	22	21	20	19	18	17	17	16	15	14	14	13	13	7s 12
48	25	24	23	21	20	19	18	17	17	16	15	14	14	13	13	12	7s 8
46	24	23	22	20	19	18	18	17	16	15	15	14	13	13	12	12	7s 3
44	23	22	21	20	19	18	17	16	15	15	14	13	13	12	12	11	6s 13
42	22	21	20	19	18	17	16	15	15	14	13	13	12	12	11	11	6s 9
40	21	20	19	18	17	16	15	15	14	13	13	12	12	11	10	10	6s 4
38	20	19	18	17	16	15	14	14	13	13	12	11	11	11	10	10	6s
36	19	18	17	16	15	14	14	13	12	12	11	11	10	10	9	9	5s 9
	4'6½	4'8	4'9½	4'11	5'½	5'2	5'4	5'5½	5'7	5'8½	5'10	5'11½	6'1	6'3	6'4½	6'6	

weight (kg)   height (ft/in)   weight (st/lbs)

Appendix

Interpreting BMI

A BMI of 18.5 to 24.9 is considered to be within the healthy weight range. Those with a BMI below 18.5 are considered underweight and at an increased health risk. A BMI of 25 to 29.9 is considered overweight. Obesity is generally defined as a BMI of greater than 30, with severe obesity being greater than 35 and morbid or extreme obesity greater than 40. Research suggests that those with a BMI of 19 to 22 enjoy the greatest longevity.

BMI does not factor in muscle mass, so very muscular people will have a high BMI, but could have a very low percentage body fat (thus, they appear 'overweight' according to BMI, but are actually very lean). In addition, very short people (less than 1.52m/5 feet tall) may have a higher BMI than would be expected relative to their size. BMI is not useful for pregnant women or those over the age of sixty-five.

The International Classification of adult underweight, overweight and obesity according to BMI (WHO 2013)

Classification	BMI (kg/m^2)
Underweight	Less than 18.50
Severe thinness	Less than 16.00
Moderate thinness	16.00 – 16.99
Mild thinness	17.00 – 18.49
Normal range	18.50 – 24.99
Overweight	More than 24.99
Pre-obese	25.00 – 29.99
Obese	More than 29.99
Obese class I	30.00 – 34.99
Obese class II	35.00 – 39.99
Obese class III	More than 39.99

Note: researchers at Oxford University's Mathematical Institute have updated the body mass index with a new formula that they say more accurately estimates body fat. The result of the change is that shorter people under 1.52m (5 feet) might gain a BMI point, while taller individuals over 1.82m (6 feet) could lose one.[1] Here's the updated calculator at Oxford University's website in which you can simply type in your height and weight: http://people.maths.ox.ac.uk/trefethen/bmi_calc.html.

Calculating Your Waist-to-Hip Ratio (WHR)

To calculate your WHR, simply:

- Measure your hips.
- Measure your waist. (To find your true waist, feel for your hip bone on one side, then move upwards until you can feel your bottom rib. Halfway between the two is your waist – for most people it is where their belly button is.)
- Divide the waist measurement by the hip measurement.

A ratio of 0.80 or less for women is considered a pear shape. A ratio of 0.85 or more in women indicates that you are carrying too much weight around your middle (apple shape), which may put you at increased risk of diseases that are linked to obesity. However, whether you are an apple or a pear may not be significant unless you are overweight according to your BMI. If you *are* overweight or obese, having an apple shape puts you at much higher risk for heart disease, type-2 diabetes, hypertension and several types of cancer. For those who naturally become apple shaped with weight gain, it is critically important that a healthy body weight be maintained.

Percentage Body Fat

Once you have a good estimate of your percentage body fat (see p. 35), check your numbers against the table below.

Percentage Body Fat

Body Type	Female
Athlete	<17%
Lean	17–22%
Normal	22–25%
Above Average	25–29%
Overfat	29–35%
Obese	35+%

This area of medicine is still undecided in terms of exactly how much fat is or isn't a risk. However, some researchers now believe that women who fall within the normal range for BMI (18.5–24.9), yet are made up of more than 30 per cent body fat are at greater health risk.[2]

References

Chapter 1

1. S. Hayes, S. Tantleff-Dunn, 'Am I too fat to be a princess? Examining the effects of popular children's media on young girls' body image', *British Journal of Developmental Psychology*, volume 28, issue 2, pp. 413–426, 2010.

2. Trisha A. Pruis, Jeri S. Janowsky, (2010) 'Assessment of Body Image in Younger and Older Women', *The Journal of General Psychology*, volume 137, issue 3, pp. 225–238, 2010, DOI: 10.1080/00221309.2010.484446; C. D. Runfola, A. Von Holle, S. E.Trace, K. A. Brownley, S. M. Hofmeier, D. A. Gagne and C. M. Bulik (2013), 'Body Dissatisfaction in Women Across the Lifespan: Results of the UNC-*SELF* and Gender and Body Image (GABI) Studies', *European Eating Disorders Review*, volume 21, issue 52–59, 2013, DOI: 10.1002/erv.2201.

3. Danielle A. Gagne, et al., 'Eating disorder symptoms and weight and shape concerns in a large web-based convenience sample of women ages 50 and above: Results of the gender and body image (GABI) study', *International Journal of Eating Disorders*, 21 June 2012, DOI: 10.1002/eat.22030.

4. Advisory Council on the Misuse of Drugs (ACMD), 'Consideration of the Anabolic Steroids', September 2010; J. O'Dea, et al., 'Nutritional supplements and weight gain behaviours in male adolescents from 2000–2010: implications for anti-doping inter-ventions and school education', ongoing study, University of Sydney, 2013.

5. V. Swami, et al., 'The Attractive Female Body Weight and Female

References

Body Dissatisfaction in 26 Countries Across 10 World Regions: Results of the International Body Project I', *Personality and Social Psychology Bulletin*, volume 36, pp. 309–325, March 2010, DOI: 10.1177/0146167209359702.

6. H. A. Sabah, et al., 'Body weight dissatisfaction and communication with parents among adolescents in 24 countries: international cross-sectional survey'. *BMC Public Health*, volume 9, issue 52, 2009, DOI: 10.1186/1471-2458-9-52.

7. Eva Wiseman, 'Uncomfortable in our skin: the body-image report', *Observer*, 10 June 2012.

8. C. Shaban (2010), 'Body image, intimacy and diabetes', *European Diabetes Nursing*, volume 7, issue 82–86, 2010, DOI: 10.1002/edn.163.

9. Dave Dhaval, Rashad Inas, 'Overweight status, self-perception, and suicidal behaviors among adolescents', *Social Science & Medicine*, volume 68, issue 9, pp. 1685–1691, May 2009, ISSN 0277-9536, http://dx.doi.org/10.1016/j.socscimed.2009.02.015.

10. R. C. Plotnikoff, et al., 'Testing a conceptual model related to weight perceptions, physical activity and smoking in adolescents', Health Education Research, volume 22, issue 2, pp. 192–202, 2007.

11. J. A. Fulkerson, S.A. French, 'Cigarette smoking for weight loss or control among adolescents: gender and racial/ethnic differences', *Journal of Adolescent Health*, volume 32, issue 4, pp. 306–13, May 2003, DOI: 10.1016/S1054-139X(02)00566-9.

12. K. Honjo, M. Siegel, 'Perceived importance of being thin and smoking initiation among young girls', *Tobacco Control*, volume 12, issue 3, pp. 289–295, September 2003, DOI: 10.1136/tc.12.3.289.

13. M. Granner, et al., (2002) 'Levels of Cigarette and Alcohol Use Related to Eating-disorder Attitudes', *American Journal of Health Behavior*, volume 26, number 1, pp. 43-55(13), January 2002.

14. D. Schooler, 'Early Adolescent Body Image Predicts Subsequent Condom Use Behavior Among Girls', *Sexuality Research and Social Policy*, volume 10, issue 1, pp. 52–61, March 2013.

15. M. W. Wiederman, 'Body Image and Sexual Functioning', in *Encyclopedia of Body Image and Human Appearance*, volume 1, edited by Thomas F. Cash, pp. 148–152, San Diego, CA: Academic Press (Elsevier), 2012.

16. NHS Choices, 'Breast cancer (female) – information prescription: Preventing breast cancer' 2012.

17. MIND, 'New findings show women run scared from outdoor exercise', 23 April 2012.
18. T. Yanover, J.K. Thompson, 'Eating problems, body image disturbances, and academic achievement: preliminary evaluation of the eating and body image disturbances academic interference scale', International Journal of Eating Disorders, volume 41, issue 2, pp. 184–7, March 2008.
19. B. L. Fredrickson, et al., 'That swimsuit becomes you: Sex differences in self-objectification, restrained eating and math performance', *Journal of Personality and Social Psychology*, volume 75, issue 2, pp. 69–284, 1998; K.D. Gapinski, et al., 'Body Objectification and "Fat Talk": Effects on Emotion, Motivation, and Cognitive Performance', *Sex Roles*, volume 48, issue 9–10, pp. 377-388, 2003.
20. B. L. Fredrickson, K. Harrison, 'Throwing Like A Girl: Self-Objectification Predicts Adolescent Girls' Motor Performance', *Journal of Sport & Social Issues*, volume 29, number 1, pp. 79–101, February 2005, DOI: 10.1177/0193723504269878.
21. K.D. Gapinsky, 2003, op. cit.
22. C. Heldman, 'Out of Body Image', *Ms Magazine*, Spring 2008; C. Heldman, M. Cahill, 'The Beast of Beauty Culture: An Analysis of the Political Effects of Self-Objectification' Western Political Science Association conference, Las Vegas, 8–10 March 2007.
23. R. M. Calogero, 'Objects Don't Object: Evidence That Self-Objectification Disrupts Women's Social Activism', *Psychological Science*, volume 24, pp. 312–318, first published on 22 January 2013, DOI: 10.1177/0956797612452574.
24. L. Pamies-Aubalat, et al., 'Adaptation and validation of the Spanish version of the Dieting Peer Competitiveness Scale to adolescents of both genders', *Journal of Health Psychology*, volume 18, pp. 1562–1571, December 2013, first published on 8 January 2013, DOI: 10.1177/1359105312465914.
25. T. F. Cash, et al., (2004) 'Body Image in an Interpersonal Context: Adult Attachment, Fear of Intimacy and Social Anxiety', *Journal of Social and Clinical Psychology*, volume 23, special issue: *Body Image and Eating Disorders: Influence of Media Images*, pp. 89–103, 2004, DOI: 10.1521/jscp.23.1.89.26987.
26. D. T. Sanchez, A.K. Kiefer (2007) 'Body concerns in and out of the bedroom: implications for sexual pleasure and problems', *Archives of Sexual Behaviour*, volume 36, issue 6, pp. 808–820, December 2007.
27. M. Meana, S. E. Nunnink (2006) 'Gender differences in the

content of cognitive distraction during sex', *Journal of Sex Research*, volume 43, issue 1, pp. 59–67, February 2006.

28. N. L. Dove, M.W. Wiederman, 'Cognitive Distraction and Women's Sexual Functioning', *Journal of Sex & Marital Therapy*, volume 26, pp. 67–78, 2000.

29. D. M. Ackard, et al., 'Effect of body image and self-image on women's sexual behaviors', *International Journal of Eating Disorders*, volume 28, issue 4, pp. 422–9, 2000.

30. L. Woertman, F. van den Brink, 'Body Image and Female Sexual Functioning and Behavior: A Review', *Journal of Sex Research*, volume 49, number 2–3, 2012.

31. A. D. Weaver, E. S. Byers, 'The relationships among body image, body mass index, exercise, and sexual functioning in heterosexual women', *Psychology of Women Quarterly*, volume 30, pp. 333–339, 2006, DOI: 10.1111/j.1471-6402.2006.00308.x.

32. B. N. Seal, et al., (2009) 'The Association Between Body Esteem and Sexual Desire Among College Women', Archives of Sexual Behaviour, volume 38, issue 5, pp. 866–872, October 2009, DOI: 10.1007/s10508-008-9467-1.

33. M. E. Munoz, C. J. Ferguson, 'Body Dissatisfaction Correlates With Inter-Peer Competitiveness, Not Media Exposure: A Brief Report', *Journal of Social and Clinical Psychology*, volume 31, number 4, pp. 383-392, 2012.

34. C. N. Markey, P. M. Markey, 'Weight Disparities Between Female Same-Sex Romantic Partners and Weight Concerns: Examining Partner Comparison', *Psychology of Women Quarterly*, volume 37, pp. 469–477, December 2013, DOI: 10.1177/0361684313484128; C. N. Markey, P. M. Markey, 'Gender, sexual orientation, and romantic partner influence on body image: An examination of heterosexual and lesbian women and their partners', *Journal of Social and Personal Relationships*, 31 May 2013, DOI: 10.1177/0265407513489472.

35. M. A. Morrison, et al., 2004. 'Does body satisfaction differ between gay men and lesbian women and heterosexual men and women?: A meta-analytic review', *Body Image*, volume 1, issue 2, pp. 127–138, May 2004; C. N. Markey, P. M. Markey, 31 May 2013, ibid.

36. M. E. Costa-Font, C. J. Jofre-Bonet, 'Body Dissatisfaction Correlates With Inter-Peer Competitiveness, Not Media Exposure: A Brief Report',' *Journal of Social and Clinical Psychology*, volume 31, number 4, pp. 383-392, 2012.

37. L. Wasylkiw, M. Williamson, 'Actual reports and perceptions of body image concerns of young women and their friends', *Sex Roles*, 2012 DOI: 10.1007/s11199-012-0227-2.

38. Rachel H. Salk, Renee Engeln-Maddox, '"If You're Fat, Then I'm Humongous!": Frequency, Content, and Impact of Fat Talk Among College Women', *Psychology of Women Quarterly*, volume 35, issue 18, 2011, DOI: 10.1177/0361684310384107.

39. H. Sharpe, U. Naumann, J. Treasure, U. Schmidt, (2013), 'Is fat talking a causal risk factor for body dissatisfaction? A systematic review and meta-analysis', *International Journal of Eating Disorders*, 2013, DOI: 10.1002/eat.22151.

40. Melissa J. Kaminski, Robert G. Magee, 'Does this book make me look fat? The effect of protagonist body weight and body esteem on female readers' body esteem', *Body Image*, volume 10, issue 2, pp. 255-258, March 2013, ISSN 1740-1445, http://dx.doi.org/10.1016/j.bodyim.2012.10.009.

41. Chapter: 'Feeding and Eating Disorders', *Diagnostic and Statistical Manual of Mental Disorders Fifth Edition*, American Psychiatric Association, 2013.

42. Royal College of Psychiatrists, Academy of Medical Royal Colleges, 'No Health without Mental Health: The supporting evidence', 2011.

43. American Psychological Association, 'New solutions: Psychologists are developing promising new treatments and conducting novel research to combat eating disorders' *Monitor* Staff, volume 40, number 4, p. 46, 2009.

44. Department of Mental Health, South Carolina, 'Eating Disorder Statistics', www.state.sc.us/dmh/anorexia/statistics.htm, 2006.

45. J. Arcelus, A. J. Mitchell, J. Wales, S. Nielsen, 'Mortality Rates in Patients With Anorexia Nervosa and Other Eating Disorders: A Meta-analysis of 36 Studies'. *Archives of General Psychiatry*, volume 68, issue 7, pp. 724–731, 2011, DOI: 10.1001/archgenpsychiatry.2011.74.

46. BEAT, 'Facts and Figures' www.b-eat.co.uk/about-beat/media-centre/facts-and-figures/, 2013; National Institute for Health and Clinical Excellence, 'Eating Disorders: National Clinical Practice Guideline CG9', 2004.

47. Crown Prosecution Service, (2011) 'Domestic Violence: the facts, the issues, the future', speech by the Director of Public Prosecutions, Keir Starmer QC, www.cps.gov.uk/news/articles/domestic_violence_-_the_facts_the_issues_the_future, 4 December 2011; Public

References

Health England, 'Deaths in 2012 among females living with HIV in the UK (≥15 years of age at death, non-black African ethnicity, heterosexual acquisition): 26 deaths', data provided by HIV/AIDS New Diagnosis team, 2013.

48. 'Faces of the Fallen. Casualties, Afghanistan', *Washington Post*, 2013, apps.washingtonpost.com/national/fallen/theaters/afghanistan/, accessed 6 June 2013.

49. B. Pavlova, et al., 'Trends in hospital admissions for eating disorders in a country undergoing a socio-cultural transition, the Czech Republic 1981-2005', *Social Psychiatry and Psychiatric Epidemiology*, volume 45, issue 5, pp. 541–550, May 2010, DOI: 10.1007/s00127-009-0092-7.

50. J. Tong, et al., 'A two-stage epidemiologic study on prevalence of eating disorders in female university students in Wuhan, China', *Social Psychiatry and Psychiatric Epidemiology*, June 2013, DOI: 10.1007/s00127-013-0694-y.

51. N. Chisuwa, J. A. O'Dea (2010). 'Body image and eating disorders among Japanese adolescents: A review of the literature' *Appetite*, volume 54, issue 1, pp. 5–15, February 2010, DOI: 10.1016/j.appet.2009.11.008.

52. T. D. Wade, M. Tiggemann, 'The role of perfectionism in body dissatisfaction', *Journal of Eating Disorders*, volume 1, issue 2, 2013, DOI: 10.1186/2050-2974-1-2.

53. S. Baron-Cohen, et al., 'Do girls with anorexia nervosa have elevated autistic traits?', *Molecular Autism*, volume 4, issue 24, 2013, DOI: 10.1186/2040-2392-4-24.

54. US Department of Health, Office on Women's Health, 'Body Image: Eating disorders', 2010.

55. Carre Otis, 'The Truth About Skinny Models', Vogue Australia, September Issue 2013.

56. M. E. Costa-Font, C. J. Jofre-Bonet, 2013, op. cit.

57. April R. Smith, Norman Li, Thomas E. Joiner, 'The Pursuit of Success: Can Status Aspirations Negatively Affect Body Satisfaction?', *Journal of Social and Clinical Psychology*, volume 30, number 5, pp. 531-547, 2011, DOI: 10.1521/jscp.2011.30.5.531.

58. E. M. Ashikali, H. Dittmar, 'The effect of priming materialism on women's responses to thin-ideal media', *British Journal of Social Psychology*, volume 51, pp. 514–533, 2012, DOI: 10.1111/j.2044-8309.2011.02020.x.

59. J. A. Boyce, et al., 'Preliminary support for links between media body ideal insecurity and women's shoe and handbag purchases',

Body Image, volume 9, issue 3, pp. 413–416, June 2012, ISSN 1740-1445, dx.doi.org/10.1016/j.bodyim.2012. 03.001.

60. K. Durkin, et al., 'The effect of images of thin and overweight body shapes on women's ambivalence towards chocolate', *Appetite*, volume 58, issue 1, pp. 222–226, February 2012, DOI: 10.1016/j.appet. 2011.09.027.

61. M. V. Day, D. R. Bobocel, 'The Weight of a Guilty Conscience: Subjective Body Weight as an Embodiment of Guilt', *PLoS ONE*, volume 8, issue 7, e69546, DOI: 10.1371/ journal.pone.0069546.

Chapter 2

1. B. W. Parks, et al., 'Genetic Control of Obesity and Gut Microbiota Composition in Response to High-Fat, High-Sucrose Diet in Mice', *Cell Metabolism*, 2013, dx.doi.org/10.1016/ j.cmet.2012.12.007.

2. 'Fat Genes' Determine Obesity, UCLA Study Says, In Addition To Diet And Exercise' *Huffington Post*, 1 October 2013.

3. Sonja Entringer, Claudia Buss, James M. Swanson, et al., 'Fetal Programming of Body Composition, Obesity, and Metabolic Function: The Role of Intrauterine Stress and Stress Biology', *Journal of Nutrition and Metabolism*, volume 2012, Article ID 632548, 16 pages, 2012, DOI: 10.1155/2012/632548.

4. B. H. Wrotniak, J. Shults, S. Butts, et al., 'Gestational weight gain and risk of overweight in the offspring at age 7 in a multi-center, multiethnic cohort study' *The American Journal of Clinical Nutrition*, volume 87, issue 6, pp. 1818–1824, 2008; A.M. Siega-Riz, A. H. Herring, K. Carrier, et al., (2010) 'Sociodemographic, perinatal, behavioral, and psychosocial pre-dictors of weight retention at 3 and 12 months postpartum' *Obesity (Silver Spring)*, volume 18, issue 10, pp. 1996–2003, 2010; L. Schack-Nielsen, K. F. Michaelsen, M. Gamborg, et al., (2010) 'Gestational weight gain in relation to offspring body mass index and obesity from infancy through adulthood', *International Journal of Obesity*, volume 34, issue 1, pp. 67–74, 2010.

5. Gregory A. Dunn, Tracy L. Bale, 'Maternal High-Fat Diet Effects on Third-Generation Female Body Size via the Paternal Lineage', *Endocrinology*, volume 152, issue 6, pp. 2228–2236, June 2011,

References

DOI: 10.1210/en.2010-1461.

6. C. H. Llewellyn, et al., 'Nature and nurture in infant appetite: analysis of the Gemini twin birth cohort', *American Journal of Clinical Nutrition*, volume 91, issue 5, pp. 1172–1179, May 2010, DOI: 10.3945/ajcn.2009.28868.

7. E. Karra, et al., 'A link between FTO, ghrelin, and impaired brain food-cue responsively', *Journal of Clinical Investigation*, volume 123, issue 8, pp. 3539–3551, 2013, DOI: 10.1172/JCI44403.

8. A. Fisher, C. H. M van Jaarsveld, C. H. Llewellyn, J. Wardle, 'Environmental Influences on Children's Physical Activity: Quantitative Estimates Using a Twin Design', *PLoS ONE*, volume 5, issue 4, E10110, 2010, DOI: 10.1371/journal.pone.0010110.

9. M. J. Muller, et al., 'Is there evidence for a set point that regulates human body weight?', *F1000 Medicine Report*, volume 2, issue 59, 2010, DOI: 10.3410/M2-59.

10. M. J. Muller, et al.,2010, op. cit.

11. K. N. Manolopoulos, et al., 'Gluteofemoral body fat as a determinant of metabolic health', *International Journal of Obesity* (London), volume 34, issue 6, pp. 949–959, June 2010, DOI: 10.1038/ijo.2009.286.

12. M.C. Zillikens, et al., 'Sex-specific genetic effects influence variation in body composition', *Diabetologia*, volume 51, pp. 2233–2241, 2008, DOI: 10.1007/s00125-008-1163-0.

13. C. Malis, et al., 'Total and regional fat distribution is strongly influenced by genetic factors in young and elderly twins', *Obesity Research*, volume 13, issue 12, pp.2139–2145, December 2006.

14. M. W. Peeters, et al., 'Genetic and environmental determination of tracking in subcutaneous fat distribution during adolescence', *American Journal of Clinical Nutrition*, volume 86, number 3, pp. 652–660, September 2007.

15. M. A. Stults-Kolehmainen, et al., 'Fat in Android, Trunk, and Peripheral Regions Varies by Ethnicity and Race in College Aged Women', *Obesity*, volume 20, pp. 660–665, 2012, DOI: 10.1038/oby.2011.300.

16. L. P. Kozak, 'The Genetics of Brown Adipocyte Induction in White Fat Depots', *Frontiers in Endocrinology*, volume 2, issue 64, 2011, DOI: 10.3389/fendo.2011.00064; P. Seale, 'Brown adipose tissue biology and therapeutic potential', *Frontiers in Endocrinology*, volume 4, issue 14, 2013, DOI: 10.3389/fendo.2013.00014.

17. S. Sullivan, et al., 'Personality characteristics in obesity and

relationship with successful weight loss', *International Journal of Obesity*, volume 31, pp. 669–674, 2007.

18. A. R. Sutin, et al., 'Personality and obesity across the adult life span', *Journal of Personality and Social Psychology*, volume 101, issue 3, pp. 579–592, September 2011.

19. M. Gambacciani, et al., 'Prospective evaluation of body weight and body fat distribution in early postmenopausal women with and without hormonal replacement therapy', *Maturitas*, volume 39, issue 2, pp.125–132, 25 August 2001

20. Harvard School of Public Health, 'How to Get to Your Healthy Weight', *The Nutrition Source*, 2013.

21. Harvard School of Public Health, 'Measuring Obesity', *Obesity Prevention Source*, 2013; Harvard School of Public Health, 'Healthy Weight', *The Nutrition Source*, 2013.

22. A. Oreopoulos, et al., 'More on Body Fat Cutoff Points–Reply–I', *Mayo Clinic Proceedings*, volume 86, issue 6, pp. 584–585, June 2011, DOI: 10.4065/mcp.2011.0156.

23. International Olympic Committee Medical Commission, 'Position stand on the female athlete triad', 2006.

24. J. M. Thein-Nissenbaum. K. E. Carr, 'Female athlete triad syndrome in the high school athlete', *Physical Therapy in Sport*, volume 12, issue 3, pp. 108–116, August 2011, DOI: 10.1016/j.ptsp.2011.04.002.

25. M. K. Torstveit, J. Sundgot-Borge, 'The female athlete triad exists in both elite athletes and controls', *Medicine and Science in Sports and Exercise*, volume 37, issue 9, pp. 1449–59, September 2005.

26. J. M. Thein-Nissenbaum, K. E. Carr 'Long term consequences of the female athlete triad', *Maturitas*, volume 72, issue 2, pp. 107–112, June 2013, DOI: 10.1016/j.maturitas.2013.02.010.

27. C. L. S. Lim, et al., 'The Body Dissatisfaction among Female Athletes and Non-athletes', *Journal of Asia Pacific Studies*, volume 2, number 1, pp. 55–69, 2011.

28. P. Cottone, et al., 'CRF system recruitment mediates dark side of compulsive eating', *Proceedings of National Academy of Sciences*, volume 106, issue 47, pp. 20016–20020, 2009.

29. M. E. Waring, et al., 'Weight cycling and overall weight status during middle age and incident cardiovascular disease events and all-cause and cardiovascular mortality'. EPI|NPAM 2010, 3 March 2010, San Francisco, CA. Abstract P138.

30. E. V. Carraça, et al., 'Body image change and improved eating

self-regulation in a weight management intervention in women', *International Journal of Behavioral Nutrition and Physical Activity*, volume 8, issue 75, 2011, DOI: 10.1186/1479-5868-8-75.

31. D. Neel, 'A "Wicked Problem": Combating Obesity in the Developing World' *Harvard College Global Health Review*, 19 October 2011.

32. S. L. Gortmaker, et al., 'Obesity 4: Changing the future of obesity: science, policy, and action', *Lancet*, volume 378, pp. 838–47, 2011.

33. J. Guthman, 'Teaching the Politics of Obesity: Insights into Neoliberal Embodiment and Contemporary Biopolitics', Antipode, volume 41, number 5, pp. 1110–11332009, ISSN 0066-4812, DOI: 10.1111/j.1467-8330.2009.00707.x.

Chapter 3

1. D. Baker, 'Body image dissatisfaction and eating attitudes in visually impaired women', *International Journal of Eating Disorders*, volume 24, issue 3, pp. 319–322, November 1998.

2. Eleni-Marina Ashikali, Helga Dittmar, 'Body image and restrained eating in blind and sighted women: A preliminary study', *Body Image*, volume 7, issue 2, pp. 172–175, 2010, ISSN 1740-1445.

3. A. E. Becker, et al., 'Eating behaviours and attitudes following prolonged exposure to television among ethnic Fijian adolescent girls', *British Journal of Psychiatry*, volume 180, pp. 509–14, 2002.

4. M. Nouri, et al., 'Media exposure, internalization of the thin ideal, and body dissatisfaction: comparing Asian American and European American college females', *Body Image*, volume 8, issue 4, pp. 366–372, September 2011, DOI: 10.1016/j.bodyim.2011.05.008.

5. E. Poloskov, T. J. Tracey, 'Internalization of U.S. female beauty standards as a mediator of the relationship between Mexican American women's acculturation and body dissatisfaction' *Body Image*, volume 10, issue 4, pp. 501–508, September 2013, first published online 25 June 2013, DOI: 10.1016/j.bodyim.2013.05.005.

6. 'Underweight models go out with 2012', *The Times of Israel*, 1 January 2013.

7. H. A. Hausenblas, et al., 'Media effects of experimental presentation of the ideal physique on eating disorder symptoms: A

meta-analysis of laboratory studies', *Clinical Psychology Review*, volume 33, pp. 168–181, 2013.

8. K. Homan, et al., 'The effect of viewing ultra-fit images on college women's body dissatisfaction', *Body Image*, volume 9, issue 1, pp. 50–56, January 2012, DOI: 10.1016/j.bodyim.2011.07.006.

9. S. Knobloch-Westerwick, J. Crane, 'A Losing Battle: Effects of Prolonged Exposure to Thin-Ideal Images on Dieting and Body Satisfaction', *Communication Research*, volume 39, p. 79, 2012, DOI: 10.1177/0093650211400596.

10. F. Wan, et al., 'The moderating role of mode of exposure', *Organizational Behavior and Human Decision Processes*, volume 120, issue 1, pp. 37–46, January 2013, doi.org/10.1016/ j.obhdp.2012.07.008.

11. A. F. Young, et al., 'The Skinny on Celebrities: Parasocial Relationships Moderate the Effects of Thin Media Figures on Women's Body Image', *Social Psychological and Personality Science*, volume 3, pp. 659-666, November 2012, first published on 2 February 2012, DOI: 10.1177/1948550611434785.

12. R. Owen, R. M. Spencer, 'Body ideals in women after viewing images of typical and healthy weight models', *Body Image*, volume 10, issue 4, pp. 489–494, September 2013, first published online on 27 May 2013, DOI: 10.1016/j.bodyim.2013.04.005.

13. A. Greene, '15 Most Bizarre Diets in History', *Yahoo Shine*, 11 May 2010.

14. S. L., Franzoi, et al., 'Exploring Body Comparison Tendencies: Women Are Self-Critical Whereas Men Are Self-Hopeful', *Psychology of Women Quarterly*, volume 36, pp. 99–109, March 2012, DOI: 10.1177/0361684311427028.

15. R. Miyamoto, Y. Kikuchi, 'Gender Differences of Brain Activity in the Conflicts Based on Implicit Self-Esteem', *PLoS ONE*, volume 7, issue 5, 2012, DOI: 10.1371/journal.pone.0037901.

16. R. Uher, et al., 'Functional neuroanatomy of body shape perception in healthy and eating disordered women', *Biological Psychiatry*, volume 58, pp. 990–997, 2005.

17. H. C. Friederich, et al., 'I'm not as slim as that girl: Neural bases of body shape self-comparison to media images', *NeuroImage*, volume 37, pp. 674–681, 2007.

18. M. Kurosaki, et al., 'Distorted images of one's own body activates the prefrontal cortex and limbic/paralimbic system in young women: a functional magnetic resonance imaging study', *Biological Psychiatry*, volume 59, issue 4, pp. 380–386, 15 February 2006, first published online on 13 September 2005.

19. Y. Miyake, et al., 'Brain activation during the perception of distorted body images in eating disorders', *Psychiatry Research: Neuroimaging*, volume 181, issue 3, pp. 183–192, 2010.

20. T. E. Owens, M. D. Allen, D. L. Spanglera, 'An fMRI study of self-reflection about body image: Sex differences', *Personality and Individual Differences*, volume 48, issue 7, pp. 849–854, 2010.

21. N. Shirao, et al., 'Gender differences in brain activity generated by unpleasant word stimuli concerning body image: an fMRI study', *British Journal of Psychiatry*, volume 186, pp. 48–53, 2005.

22. C. Herbert, et al., 'Risk for Eating Disorders Modulates Startle Responses to Body Words', *PLoS ONE*, volume 8, issue 1, 2013, DOI: 10.1371/journal.pone.0053667.

23. G. S. O'Keeffe, K. Clarke-Pearson, 'AAP Council On Communications And Media. Clinical Report – The Impact of Social Media on Children, Adolescents, and Families', *Pediatrics*, volume 127, issue 4, pp. 799–804, 2011, DOI: 10.1542/peds.2011-0054.

24. A. Sigman, (2012) 'Time for a view on screen time', *Archives of Disease in Childhood*, volume 97, issue 11, pp. 935–942, 2012, DOI: 10.1136/archdischild-2012-302196.

25. S. E. Gutierres, et al., 'Beauty, Dominance, and the Mating Game: Contrast Effects in Self-Assessment Reflect Gender Differences in Mate Selection', *Personality and Social Psychology Bulletin*, volume 25, issue 9, pp. 1126–1134, 1999.

25. R. Quian Quiroga, 'Searching for the Jennifer Aniston Neuron', *Scientific American*, 18 January 2013.

26. T. Northup, 'Triggering Body Dissatisfaction: The Role of Familiarity on Subsequent Evaluations of the Self', *Journalism and Mass Communication*, volume 2, number 1, pp. 294–303, 2012.

Chapter 4

1. Centers for Disease Control and Prevention, 'Reproductive Health: Maternal and Infant Health', 2013; B. Hill, et al., 'Body Image and Gestational Weight Gain: A Prospective Study', *Journal of Midwifery & Women's Health*, volume 58, pp. 189–194, 2013, DOI: 10.1111/j.1542-2011.2012.00227.x.

2. National Institute for Health and Care Excellence, 'NICE issues pregnancy weight management guidance, as the number of obese mothers soars', news statement, 28 July 2010.

3. K. D. Suschinsky, M. L. Lalumière, 'Is sexual concordance related to awareness of physiological states?', *Archives of Sexual Behaviour*, volume 41, issue 1, pp. 199–208, 2012, DOI: 10.1007/s10508-012-9931-9.

4. M. L. Chivers, et al., 'Gender and Sexual Orientation Differences in Sexual Response to Sexual Activities Versus Gender of Actors in Sexual Films', *Journal of Personality and Social Psychology*, volume 93, number 6, pp. 1108–1121, 2007, DOI: 10.1037/0022-3514.93.6.1108.

5. R. Blanchard, et al., 'Sexual Attraction to Others: A Comparison of Two Models of Alloerotic Responding in Men', *Archives of Sexual Behaviour*, volume 41, pp. 13–29, 2012, DOI 10.1007/s10508-010-9675-3.

6. P. Fromberger, et al., 'Initial Orienting Towards Sexually Relevant Stimuli: Preliminary Evidence from Eye Movement Measures', *Archives of Sexual Behaviour*, volume 41, pp. 919–928, 2012, DOI 10.1007/s10508-011-9816-3.

7. J. C. Karremans, et al., 'Blind men prefer a low waist-to-hip ratio', *Evolution and Human Behavior*, volume 31, pp. 182–186, 2010.

8. F. Pazhoohi, J. R. Liddle, 'Identifying feminine and masculine ranges for waist-to-hip ratio', *Journal of Social, Evolutionary, and Cultural Psychology*, volume 6, issue 2, pp. 227–232, 2012.

9. F. Pazhoohi, et al., 'Iranian Men's Waist-To-Hip Ratios, Shoulder-To-Hip Ratios, Body Esteem And Self-Efficacy', *Journal of Evolutionary Psychology*, pp. 61–67, 2012, DOI: 10.1556/ JEP.10.2012.2.2.

10. D. Singh, et al., 'Did the perils of abdominal obesity affect depiction of feminine beauty in the sixteenth to eighteenth century British literature? Exploring the health and beauty link', *Proceeding of the Royal Society B*, volume 274 pp. 891–894, 2007.

11. D. Lassek, J. C. Gaulin, 'Waist-hip ratio and cognitive ability: is gluteofemoral fat a privileged store of neurodevelopmental resources?' *Evolution and Human Behavior*, volume 29, pp. 26–34, 2008.

12. J. A. Bremser, G. G. Gallup, 'Mental State Attribution and Body Configuration in Women', Frontiers in Evolutionary Neuroscience, volume 4, issue 1, 2012, DOI: 10.3389/fnevo. 2012.00001

References

13. J. Kosiak, 'Body image in homosexual persons', *Psychiatria Polska,* volume 43, issue 1, pp. 99–107, Jan–Feb 2009.

14. A. B. Cohen, I.J. Tannenbaum, 'Lesbian and bisexual women's judgments of the attractiveness of different body types', *Journal Of Sex Research*, volume 38, issue 3, pp. 226–232, 2001.

15. Viren Swami, Martin J. Tovée, 'The Influence of Body Mass Index on the Physical Attractiveness Preferences of Feminist and Nonfeminist Heterosexual Women and Lesbians', *Psychology of Women Quarterly*, volume 20, pp. 252–257, September 2006, DOI: 10.1111/j.1471-6402.2006.00293.x.

16. C.J. Huxley, et al., '"It's a Comparison Thing, Isn't It?": Lesbian and Bisexual Women's Accounts of How Partner Relationships Shape Their Feelings About Their Body and Appearance', *Psychology of Women Quarterly*, volume 35, pp. 415–427, September 2011, DOI: 10.1177/0361684311410209.

17. A. Furnham, V. Swami, 'Perception of female buttocks and breast size in profile', *Social Behavior And Personality*, volume 35, issue 1, pp.1–8, 2007.

18. B. Dagnino. J. Navajas, M. Sigman, 'Eye Fixations Indicate Men's Preference for Female Breasts or Buttocks', *Archives of Sexual Behaviour*, volume 41, issue 4, pp. 929–937, 2012.

19. F. Marlowe, et al., 'Men's preferences for women's profile waist-to-hip ratio in two societies', *Evolution and Human Behaviour*, volume 26, pp. 458–468, 2005.

20. V. Swami, M. J. Tovee, 'The Impact of Psychological Stress on Men's Judgements of Female Body Size', *PLoS ONE*, volume 7, issue 8, 2012, DOI: 10.1371/ journal.pone.0042593.

21. V. Swami, M. J. Tovee, 'Resource Security Impacts Men's Female Breast Size Preferences', *PLoS ONE*, volume 8, issue 3, 2013, DOI: 10.1371/journal.pone.005762.

22. O. Ogas, S. Gaddam, from authors' summary in '5 Things That Internet Porn Reveals About Our Brains', *Discover*, September 20 2011.

23. R. Blanchard, et al., 2012, op. cit.

24. Y. Xu, A. Lee, W-L. Wu, X Liu, P. Birkholz, 'Human Vocal Attractiveness as Signaled by Body Size Projection', *PLoS ONE*, volume 8, issue 4, 2013, DOI: 10.1371/journal.pone.0062397.

25. R. N. Pipitone, G. G. Gallup, 'Women's voice attractiveness varies across the menstrual cycle', *Evolution and Human Behavior*, volume 29, issue 4, pp. 268–274, 2008.

26. R. N. Pipitone, G. G. Gallup, 'The Unique Impact of Menstru-

ation on the Female Voice: Implications for the Evolution of Menstrual Cycle Cues', *Ethology*, volume 118, pp. 281–291, 2012, DOI: 10.1111/j.1439-0310.2011.02010.x.

27. Martin T. Thema, 'Side Hustle Series: I'm a "Phone Actress"', 27 October 2011, www.budgetsaresexy.com/2011/10/how-to-be-phone-sex-operator/.

28. British Association for Counselling and Psychotherapy, 2013; American Psychological Association, 'Men: A growing minority?' by Cassandra Willyard in *GradPSYCH Magazine*, 2013.

29. J. A. Hall, M. Schmid Mast, 'Are Women Always More Interpersonally Sensitive Than Men? Impact of Goals and Content Domain', Personality and Social Psychology Bulletin, volume 34, issue 1, pp. 144–155 January 2008, DOI: 10.1177/0146167207309192.

30. A. Urbanik, et al., 'Functional Magnetic Resonance Imaging of the Gender Differences in Activation of the Brain Emotional Centres', study presented at the annual meeting of the Radiological Society of North America. Session: Neuroradiology/ Head and Neck, 29 November 2009.

31. B. Fink, et al., 'Women's body movements are a potential cue to ovulation', *Personality and Individual Differences*, volume 53, issue 6, pp. 759–763, October 2012, ISSN 0191-8869, dx.doi.org/10.1016/j.paid.2012.06.005.

32. Bridget Murray Law, 'Hormones & desire', *American Psychological Association*, volume 42, number 3, March 2011.

33. 'Men look for less pretty wives', WantChinaTimes.com, 8 October 2012.

34. 'Men Puzzled By Debate Over Bouncy Girls', Daily Mash, 23 March 2010, www.thedailymash.co.uk/news/society/men-puzzled-by-debate-over-bouncy-girls-201003232584.

Chapter 5

1. J. Turner, 'Now showing: how the bump went public', *The Times*, 18 May 2013.

2. M. Fuller-Tyszkiewicz, et al., 'Body dissatisfaction during pregnancy: A systematic review of cross-sectional and prospective correlates', *Journal of Health Psychology*, volume 18, number 11, pp. 1411–1421, November 2012; A. Clark, et al., 'My baby

body: A qualitative insight into women's body related experiences and mood during pregnancy and the postpartum', *Journal of Reproductive and Infant Psychology*, volume 27, issue 4, 2009b, DOI: 10.1080/02646830903190904.

3. A. Clark, et al., 2009b ibid.

4. K. D. Mickelson, J. A. Joseph, 'Postpartum Body Satisfaction and Intimacy in First-Time Parents', *Sex Roles*, volume 67, issue 5–6, pp. 300–310, September 2012, DOI: 10.1007/s11199-012-0192-9.

5. D. Gjerdingen, et al., 'Predictors of mothers' postpartum body dissatisfaction', *Women Health,* volume 49, issue 6, pp. 491–504, 2009.

6. J. Collingwood, 'Body Dissatisfaction and Pregnancy', Psych Central, 2010, retrieved on 17 May 2013 from psychcentral.com/lib/2010/body-dissatisfaction-and-pregnancy/.

7. E.L. Rauff, D. S. Downs, 'Mediating Effects of Body Image Satisfaction on Exercise Behavior, Depressive Symptoms, and Gestational Weight Gain in Pregnancy', *Annals of Behavioral Medicine*, volume 42, issue 3, pp. 381–390, 2011.

8. A. Clark, et al., 'The relationship between depression and body dissatisfaction across pregnancy and the postpartum: a prospective study', *Journal of Health Psychology*, volume 14, number 1, pp. 23-31, 2009a; A. Clark, et al., 2009b, op. cit.

9. N. I. Gavin, et al., 'Perinatal depression: A systematic review of prevalence and incidence', *Obstetrics and Gynecology*, volume 106, issue 5, part 1, pp. 1071–1083, 2005.

10. M. Fuller-Tyszkiewicz, et al., November 2012, op. cit.

11. H. Wrotniak, J. Shults, S. Butts, et al., 2008, op. cit.; A. M. Siega-Riz, et al., 'Sociodemographic, perinatal, behavioral, and psychosocial predictors of weight retention at 3 and 12 months postpartum', *Obesity*, volume 18 issue 10, pp. 1996–2003, 2010; L. Schack-Nielsen, et al., 'Gestational weight gain in relation to offspring body mass index and obesity from infancy through adulthood', *International Journal of Obesity*, volume 34, issue 1, pp. 67–74, 2010.

12. M. Bagheri, et al., 'Pre-pregnancy Body Size Dissatisfaction and Excessive Gestational Weight Gain', *Maternal and Child Health Journal*, volume 17, issue 4, pp. 699–707, 2013; B. Hill, et al., 'Body Image and Gestational Weight Gain: A Prospective Study', *Journal of Midwifery & Women's Health*, volume 58, issue, pp.189–194, 2013.

13. M. Bagheri, et al., 2013, ibid.
14. H. Skouteris, et al., 'A prospective study of factors that lead to body dissatisfaction during pregnancy', *Body Image*, volume 2, issue 4, pp. 347–361, 2005.
15. World Health Organization, 'Exclusive breastfeeding for six months best for babies everywhere', statement, 15 January 2011; World Health Organization 'Fact Files: 10 facts on breastfeeding', July 2012.
16. I. Johnston-Robledo, V. Fred, 'Self- objectification and lower income pregnant women's breastfeeding attitudes', *Journal of Applied Social Psychology*, volume 38, issue 1, pp. 1–21, 2008.
17. Madoka Inoue, 'Breastfeeding and perceptions of breast shape changes in Australian and Japanese women', Ph.D. Curtin University, School of Public Health, 2012.
18. M. Fuller-Tyszkiewicz, et al., November 2012, op. cit.
19. H. Skouteris, et al., 2005, op. cit.
20. D. Gjerdingen, et al., 2009, op. cit.
21. J. Turner, 2013, op. cit.
22. Maureen Orth, 'Carla On a Hot Tin Roof', *Vanity Fair*, June 2013.
23. 'Radiant Jennifer Lopez back in shape just five weeks after giving birth to twins', *Mail Online*, 1 April 2008, www.dailymail.co.uk/tvshowbiz/article-549968/Radiant-Jennifer-Lopez-shape-just-weeks-giving-birth-twins.html.
24. Bonnie Rochman, 'Blue Ivy League: Beyonce and the need for more celebrities who breast-feed', *Time Magazine*, 19 March 2012.
25. A. Hjelmstedt, *In Vitro Fertilization – Emotional Reactions to Treatment, Pregnancy and Parenthood*, Karolinska University Press: Stockholm, Sweden, 2003.
26. H. Skouteris, et al., 2005, op. cit.
27. J. Collingwood, 2013, op. cit.
28. A. Hjelmstadt, 2003, op. cit.

Chapter 6

1. T. Ferriss, 'From Geek to Freak: How I Gained 34 lbs. of Muscle in 4 Weeks!', 2013, www.fourhourworkweek.com/blog/2007/04/29/from-geek-to-freak-how-i-gained-34-lbs-of-muscle-in-4-weeks/.

References

2. ZenHabits, 'How to Go From Skinny to Muscular in 7 Steps' (with a diet plan), 12 November 2007, zenhabits.net/how-to-go-from-skinny-to-muscular-in-7-steps-with-a-diet-plan/.
3. R. Breurer, 'Examining the Relationships between Recreational Physical Activity, Body Image and Sexual Functioning and Satisfaction in Men' MSc Thesis, University of Guelph, Ontario, Canada, 2013.
4. P. de Sousa, 'Body-image and obesity in adolescence: A comparative study of social- demographic, psychological and behavioural aspects', *The Spanish Journal of Psychology*, volume 11, issue 2, pp. 551–563, 2008.
5. R. Breurer, 2013, op. cit.
6. K. E. Heron, et al., 'Assessing Body Image in Young Children: A Preliminary Study of Racial and Developmental Differences', *SAGE Open*, volume 3, issue 1, February 2013, DOI: 10.1177/2158244013478013.
7. J. E. Leone, et al., 'Recognition and Treatment of Muscle Dysmorphia and Related Body Image Disorders', *Journal of Athletic Training*, volume 40, issue 4, pp. 352–359, 2005.
8. M. E. Eisenberg, et al., 'Muscle-enhancing Behaviors Among Adolescent Girls and Boys', *Pediatrics*, volume 130, issue 6, pp. 1019–1026, 2012.
9. D. A. Hargreaves, M. Tiggemann, '"Body Image Is for Girls" A Qualitative Study of Boys' Body Image', *Journal of Health Psychology*, volume 11, issue 4, pp. 567–576, 2006.
10. K. D. Krawiec, 'The effects of the mesomorphic ideal on men's body image, mood, self-esteem and muscle-building behaviour: Mechanisms of social comparison and body image investment', *Dissertation Abstracts International, Section B: Sciences and Engineering*, 2009, retrieved from search.proquest.com/docview/60369850?accountid=12763.
11. K. Harrison, B. J. Bond, 'Gaming magazines and the drive for muscularity in preadolescent boys: A longitudinal examination', *Body Image*, volume 4, 269–277, 2007, DOI: 10.1016/j.bodyim.2007.03.003.
12. N. Martins, et al., 'Virtual muscularity: A content analysis of male video game characters', *Body Image*, volume 8, pp. 43–51, 2010, DOI: 10.1016/j.bodyim.2010.10.002.
13. BBC News, 'Boys suffer poor body image, say teachers', 23 March 2013, www.bbc.co.uk/news/education-21864312.
14. M. Tiggermann, Y. Martins, L. Churchett, 'Beyond muscles.

Unexplored parts of mens' body image', *Journal of Health Psychology*, volume 13, issue 8, pp. 1163–1172, 2008, DOI: 10.1177/1359105308095971.

15. R. Breurer, 2013, op. cit.

16. P. Gontero, et al., 'A pilot phase-II prospective study to test the "efficacy" and tolerability of a penile-extender device in the treatment of "short penis"', *BJU International*, volume 103 pp. 793–797, 2009, DOI: 10.1111/j.1464-410X.2008.08083.x.

17. K. R. Wylie, I. Eardley, 'Penile size and the "small penis syndrome"', *BJU International*, volume 99, pp.1449–1455, 2007.

18. H. Son, et al., 'Studies on self-esteem of penile size in young Korean military men' *Asian Journal of Andrology*, volume 5, pp. 185–189, 5 September 2003.

19. J. Talalaj, S. Talalaj, 'The Strangest Human Sex, Ceremonies and Customs', Melbourne: Hill of Content, 1994.

20. J. Lever, D. A. Fredereicjk, L. A. Peplau, 'Does size matter? Men's and women's views on penis size across the lifespan', *Psychology of Men & Masculinity*, volume 3, pp. 129–43, 2006.

21. D. A. Frederick, D. M. T. Fesslet, M. G. Haselton, 'Do representations of male masculinity differ in men's and women's magazines?', *Body Image*, volume 2, pp. 81–6, March 2005.

22. J. Lever, D. A. Fredereicjk, L. A. Peplau, 2006, op. cit.

23. BBC News, 'Parliamentary porn consumption laid bare in official figures', 4 September 2013, www.bbc.co.uk/news/uk-politics-23954447.

24. Lever, D. A. Fredereicjk, L. A. Peplau, 2006, op. cit.

25. 'Get Great Abs', Men's Health, 2013a, accessed 17 September 2013, www.menshealth.co.uk/building-muscle/abs-workout/.

26. Advisory Council on the Misuse of Drugs (ACDM), 2010, op. cit.

27. A. Kicman, 'Anabolic steroids' hold on young men', News, King's College, School of Biomedical Sciences, 20 September 2013, www.kcl.ac.uk/biohealth/research/divisions/aes/newsevents/newsrecords/2013/Mar/Anabolic-steroids-hold-on-young-men.aspx.

28. BBC News, 'More Asian teens "using steroids"', 20 July 2009, news.bbc.co.uk/1/hi/uk/8158081.stm.

29. Centre for Public Health, 'Human Enhancement Drugs: The Emerging Challenges to Public Health', April 2012.

30. J. O'Dea, et al., 2013, op. cit.

31. National Institute on Drug Abuse (NIDA), 'Drug Facts: Anabolic

Steroids' July 2012, www.drugabuse.gov/publications/drugfacts/anabolic-steroids.

32. Sky News, 'Steroids "Put Teenage Bodybuilders At Risk"', 2013, news.sky.com/story/1101193/steroids-put-teenage-bodybuilders-at-risk.

33. 'Build an eight-pack in less time', *Men's Health*, 2013b, www.menshealth.co.uk/building-muscle/abs-workout/eight-pack-micro-workout.

34. E. Schuster, et al., 'The effects of appearance-related commentary on body dissatisfaction, eating pathology, and body change behaviors in men', *Psychology of Men & Masculinity*, volume 14, issue 1, pp. 76–87, January 2013.

35. 'Face Moisturizer Manufacturing in the US: Market Research Report', IBISWorld, 2013, www.ibisworld.com/industry/face-moisturizer- manufacturing.html.

The Shape of Things to Come

1. M. E. Costa-Font, C. J. Jofre-Bonet, 2013, op. cit.
2. S. Snapp, et al., 'A Body Image Resilience Model for First-Year College Women', *Sex Roles*, volume 67, pp. 211–221, 2012, DOI: 10.1007/s11199-012-0163-1.

Chapter 7

1. C. T. Chambers, et al., 'Psychological interventions for reducing pain and distress during routine childhood immunizations: a systematic review', Clinical Therapeutics, volume 31, supplement 2: S77-S103, 2009, DOI: 10.1016/j.clinthera.2009.07.023.

2. D. H. Bradshaw, et al., 'Individual Differences in the Effects of Music Engagement on Responses to Painful Stimulation', *Journal of Pain*, volume 12, issue 12, pp. 1262–1273, December 2011.

3. L. Hartling, A. S. Newton, Y. Liang, et al., 'Music to Reduce Pain and Distress in the Pediatric Emergency Department: A Randomized Clinical Trial', *JAMA Pediatrics*, volume 167, issue 9, pp. 826–835, 2013, DOI: 10.1001/jamapediatrics.2013.200.

4. D. Veale, R. Willson, A. Clark, *Overcoming Body Image Problems*

(including body dysmorphic disorder), Constable and Robinson, 2009.

5. J. Danckert, 'Descent of the Doldrums', *Scientific American*, July 2013.
6. R. Aird, 'New religious beliefs focus too much on self', University of Queensland, Communications, 17 January 2008, www.uq. edu.au/news/article/2008/01/new-religious-beliefs-focus-too-much-self.
7. J. Barton, J. Pretty, 'What is the Best Dose of Nature and Green Exercise for Improving Mental Health? A Multi-Study Analysis', *Environmental Science & Technology*, volume 44, issue 10, pp. 3947–3955, 2010; M. P. White, et al., 'Would You Be Happier Living in a Greener Urban Area? A Fixed-Effects Analysis of Panel Data', *Psychological Science*, volume 24, issue 12, pp. 2429–2436, December 2013.
8. F. E. Kuo, A. F. Taylor, 'A potential natural treatment for attention deficit/hyperactivity disorder: evidence from a national study', *American Journal of Public Health*, volume 94, issue 9, pp. 1580–86, 2004; A. F. Taylor and F. E. Kuo, 'Children With Attention Deficits Concentrate Better After Walk in the Park', *Journal of Attention Disorders*, volume 12, pp. 402–409, March 2009 DOI: 10.1177/1087054708323000; A. F. Taylor, F. E. Kuo, 'Could Exposure to Everyday Green Spaces Help Treat ADHD? Evidence from Children's Play Settings', *Applied Psychology: Health and Well-Being*, volume 3, issue 3, pp. 281–303, 2011.
9. N. M. Wells, G. W. Evans, 'Nearby Nature: A Buffer of Life Stress Among Rural Children', *Environment and Behavior*, volume 35, issue 3, pp. 311–330, 2003.
10. N. Weinstein, et al., 'Can Nature Make Us More Caring? Effects of Immersion in Nature on Intrinsic Aspirations and Generosity', Personality and Social Psychology Bulletin, volume 35, pp. 1315–1329, 2009, DOI: 10.1177/0146167209341649.
11. J. DeWolfe, et al., 'The Relationship between Levels of Greenery and Landscaping at Track and Field Sites, Anxiety, and Sports Performance of Collegiate Track and Field Athletes', *HortTechnology*, volume 21, number 3, pp. 329–335, June 2011.
12. J. Barton, J. Pretty, 2010, op. cit.
13. M. P. White, et al., 2013, op. cit.
14. S. Caparos, S., K. J. Linnell, J. Karina, A. J. Bremner, et al., 2013. 'Do local and global perceptual biases tell us anything about local and global selective attention?', *Psychological Science*,

volume 24, issue 2, pp. 206–212, 2013, ISSN 0956-7976.

15. J. Woo, et al., 'Green space, psychological restoration, and telomere length', *The Lancet*, volume 373, issue 9660, pp. 299–300, 2009, DOI: 10.1016/S0140-6736(09)60094-5.

16. R. M. Ryan, et al., 'Vitalizing effects of being outdoors and in nature', *Journal of Environmental Psychology*, volume 30, issue 2, pp. 159–168, June 2010, ISSN 0272-4944, http://dx.doi.org/10.1016/j.jenvp.2009.10.009.

17. P. A. Zaradic, O. R. W. Pergams, 'Videophilia: Implications for Childhood Development and Conservation', *The Journal of Developmental Processes*, volume 2, issue 1, pp. 130–144, Spring 2007.

18. C. S. Marsiglia, et al., 'Impact of Parenting Styles and Locus of Control on Emerging Adults' Psychosocial Success', *Journal of Education and Human Development*, volume 1, issue 1, 2007.

19. C. Sharp, et al., 'Facilitation of Internal Locus of Control in Adolescent Alcoholics Through a Brief Biofeedback-Assisted Autogenic Relaxation Training Procedure', *Journal of Substance Abuse Treatment*, volume 14, number 1, pp. 55–60, 1997.

20. X. Liu, et al., 'Life events, locus of control, and behavioral problems among Chinese adolescents', *Journal of Clinical Psychology*, volume 56, issue 12 , pp. 1565–1577, 2000.

21. M. Trentoa, et al., (2006) 'Evaluation of the locus of control in patients with type 2 diabetes after long-term management by group care', *Diabetes & Metabolism*, volume 32, issue 1, pp. 77–81, February 2006.

22 Australian Red Cross, 'Regional Development. 1970-1979: A Decade of Disasters' 2008a, www.redcross.org.au/nsw/4981EB607CAD47CF8FF9E0AF385C0FF1.htm; Australian Red Cross, 'Tasmania', 2008b, www.redcross.orf.au/TAS/aboutus_histTAS.htm.

23. D. S. Yeager, A. S. Miu, J. Powers, C. S. Dweck, 'Implicit theories of personality and attributions of hostile intent: A meta-analysis, an experiment, and a longitudinal intervention', *Child Development*, volume 84, issue 5, pp. 1651–1667, September–October 2013, DOI: 10.1111/cdev.12062.

24. F. D. Wolinsky, et al., 'Does cognitive training improve internal locus of control among older adults?', *The Journals of Gerontology, Series B: Psychological Sciences and Social Sciences*, volume 65, issue 5, pp. 591–598, September 2010, DOI: 10.1093/geronb/gbp117.

Chapter 8

1. H. Guiney, L. Machado, 'Benefits of regular aerobic exercise for executive functioning in healthy populations', *Psychonomic Bulletin & Review*, volume 20, issue 1, pp. 73–86, 2013.
2. Harvard Medical School, 'Special Health Report: Understanding Depression', Harvard Health Publications, accessed December 2013, www.health.harvard.edu/special_health_reports/Understanding_Depression.
3. P. Gorczynski, G. Faulkner, 'Exercise therapy for schizophrenia', *Cochrane Database of Systematic Reviews*, volume 12, issue 5, 12 May 2010, DOI: 10.1002/14651858.CD004412.pub2.
4. H. Boecker, et al., 'The Runner's High: Opioidergic Mechanisms in the Human Brain', *Cerebral Cortex*, volume 18, pp. 2523–2531, November 2008, DOI: 10.1093/cercor/bhn013.
5. D. A. Raichlen, et al., 'Exercise-induced endocannabinoid signaling is modulated by intensity', *European Journal of Applied Physiology*, volume 113, issue 4, pp. 869–875, 2013, epub 19 September 2012, DOI: 10.1007/s00421-012-2495-5.
6. Harvard Medical School, 2013, op. cit.
7. Mental Health Foundation, 'Let's Get Physical: The impact of physical activity on wellbeing', report, May 2013.
8. State Government of Victoria, 'Physical Activity: Women', 2013, www.betterhealth.vic.gov.au/bhcv2/bhcarticles.nsf/pages/Physical_activity_women.
9. Mind, 'New findings show women run scared from outdoor exercise', news statement, 23 April 2012.
10. K. Monshouwer, et al., 'Possible Mechanisms Explaining the Association Between Physical Activity and Mental Health: Findings From the 2001 Dutch Health Behaviour in School-Aged Children Survey', *Clinical Psychological Science*, first published online on 7 September 2012, DOI: 10.1177/2167702612450485.
11. D. L. Schmalz, et al., 'A Longitudinal Assessment of the Links Between Physical Activity and Self-Esteem in Early Adolescent Non-Hispanic Females, *Journal of Adolescent Health*, volume 41, issue 6, pp. 559–565, December 2007, DOI: 10.1016/j.jadohealth.2007.07.001.
12. E. McAuley, et al., 'Physical activity, self-efficacy, and self-esteem: longitudinal relationships in older adults', *The Journals of Gerontology, Series B: Psychological Sciences and Social Sciences*,

volume 60, issue 5, pp. 268–275, September 2005.

13. A. Campbell, H. A. Hausenblas, 'Effects of exercise interventions on body image: A meta-analysis', *Journal of Health Psychology*, issue 14, pp. 780–793, 2009.

14. K. A. Ginis, R. L. Bassett, *Exercise and changes in body image*, Guilford Press, 2011.

15. G. S. Goldfield, et al., 'The Effects of Aerobic Exercise on Psychosocial Functioning of Adolescents Who Are Overweight or Obese', *Journal of Pediatric Psychology*, volume 37, issue 10, pp. 1136–1147, November/December 2012, DOI: 10.1093/jpepsy/jss084.

16. H. A. Hausenblas, E. A. Fallon, 'Exercise and body image: A meta-analysis', *Psychology and Health*, volume 21 issue 1, pp. 33–47, 2006.

17. D. Symons Downs, et al., 'Determinants of Pregnancy and Postpartum Depression: Prospective Influences of Depressive Symptoms, Body Image Satisfaction, and Exercise Behavior', *Annals of Behavioral Medicine*, volume 36, issue 1, pp. 54–63, 2008.

18. Edmund O. Acevedo, *The Oxford Handbook of Exercise Psychology*, Oxford University Press, 2012.

19. Ibid.

20. British Heart Foundation, 'Physical Activity Statistics 2012', London 2012, ISBN 978-1-899088-07-2.

21. Mental Health Foundation, May 2013, op. cit.

22. P. Cagniart 2000. 'Seneca's Attitude Towards Sport and Athletics', *The American Journal of Ancient History*, volume 14, issue 4, pp. 162–170, 2000; N. S. Gill, Seneca's Healthy Mind, Healthy Body, 2013 ancienthistory.about.com/od/seneca/a/ 020210 SenecaonSportsandExercise.htm.

23. A. Vogel, 'Boosting Body Image in Your Classes', *IDEA Fitness Edge*, volume 2003, number 2, April 2002; BBC News, 'Eating disorders "prevalent among fitness professionals"', 31 December 2012, www.bbc.co.uk/news/uk-england-bristol-20338153.

24. A. Vogel, 2002, op. cit.

25. Mental Health Foundation, May 2013, op. cit.

Chapter 9

1. C. G. Jung, *Modern Man in Search of a Soul*, p. 49, *Psychology Press*, 2001.
2. V. Menon, M. Demaray, 'Child and Adolescent Social Support Scale for Healthy Behaviors: Scale Development and Assessment of the Relation Between Targeted Social Support and Body Size Dissatisfaction', *Children's Health Care*, volume 42, issue 1, 2013.
3. Department of Health, Australian Government, 'Preventing Eating Disorders', 2013, www.nedc.com.au/preventing-eating-disorders.
4. J. Holt-Lunstad, T. B. Smith, J. B. Layton, 'Social Relationships and Mortality Risk: A Meta-analytic Review', *PLoS Medicine*, volume 7, issue 7, 2010, DOI: 10.1371/journal.pmed.1000316.
5. S. W. Cole, et al., 'Social regulation of gene expression in human leukocytes', Genome Biology, volume 8, R189, 2007.
6. H. H. Fung, et al., 'Benefits of negative social exchanges for emotional closeness', *The Journals of Gerontology, Series B: Psychological Sciences and Social Sciences*, volume 64, issue 5, pp. 612–621, 2009, DOI: 10.1093/geronb/gbp065.
7. A. R. Smith, et al., 'Status Update: Maladaptive Facebook usage predicts increases in body dissatisfaction and bulimic symptoms', *Journal of Affective Disorders*, volume 149, issues 1–3, pp. 235–240, July 2013, ISSN 0165-0327, dx.doi.org/10.1016/ j.jad.2013.01.032.
8. E. Kross, P. Verduyn, E. Demiralp, J. Park, D. S. Lee, et al., 'Facebook Use Predicts Declines in Subjective Well-Being in Young Adults', *PLoS ONE*, volume 8, issue 8, 2013, DOI: 10.1371/journal.pone.0069841.
9. A. Sigman, 'Well Connected?: The Biological Implications of "Social Networking"', *The Biologist*, volume 56, issue 1, pp. 14–20, 2009.
10. N. H. Nie, et al., 'Ten years after the birth of the Internet: how do Americans use the Internet in their daily lives?', report: Stanford Institute For The Quantitative Study Of Society, Stanford University, 2005.
11. Public Health England, 'How healthy behaviour supports children's wellbeing', Crown Copyright, 28 August 2013.
12. US Department of Health and Human Services, 'Healthy People 2020, Objective PA-8: Increase the proportion of children and

adolescents who do not exceed recommended limits for screen time', 2013, healthypeople.gov/2020/.

13. L. B. Aknin, et al., 'Does Social Connection Turn Good Deeds into Good Feelings?: The Value of Putting the "Social" in Prosocial Spending', *International Journal of Happiness and Development*, volume 1, issue 2, pp. 155–171, 2013.

14. E. Kahana, et al., 'Altruism, Helping, and Volunteering: Pathways to Well-Being in Late Life', *Journal of Aging and Health*, February 2013 volume 25, pp.159–187, DOI: 10.1177/089826 4312469665.

15. S. L. Brown, et al., 'Providing Social Support May Be More Beneficial Than Receiving It: Results From a Prospective Study of Mortality', *Psychological Science*, volume 14, pp. 320–327, July 2003, DOI: 10.1111/1467-9280.14461.

16. M. J. Poulin, et al., 'Giving to Others and the Association Between Stress and Mortality', *American Journal of Public Health*, volume 103, number 9, pp. 1649–1655 September 2013, DOI: 10.2105/AJPH.2012.300876.

17. H. M. C. Schreier., et al., 'Effect of Volunteering on Risk Factors for Cardiovascular Disease in Adolescents: a Randomized Controlled Trial', *JAMA Pediatrics,* volume 167, issue 4, pp. 327–332, 2013, DOI: 10.1001/jamapediatrics.2013.1100.

18. S. Kim, K. F. Ferraro, 'Do Productive Activities Reduce Inflammation in Later Life? Multiple Roles, Frequency of Activities, and C-Reactive Protein' *The Gerontologist,* 2013, first published online on 22 August 2013, DOI: 10.1093/geront/gnt090.

19. S. A. Reid-Arndt, M. L. Smith, D. P. Yoon, B. Johnstone, 'Gender Differences in Spiritual Experiences, Religious Practices, and Congregational Support for Individuals with Significant Health Conditions', *Journal of Religion, Disability & Health*, volume 15, issue 2, pp. 175–196, 2011.

20. M. Inzlicht, et al., 'Neural Markers of Religious Conviction', *Psychological Science*, volume 20, pp. 385–392, March 2009, DOI: 10.1111/j.1467-9280.2009.02305.x.

21. K. Rounding, et al., 'Religion Replenishes Self-Control', *Psychological Science*, volume 23, issue 6, pp. 635–642, June 2012.

22. G. N. Levine, et al., 'Pet Ownership and Cardiovascular Risk: A Scientific Statement From the American Heart Association', *Circulation*, 9 May 2013 DOI: 10.1161/CIR.0b013e31829201e1.

23. S. Staats, H. Wallace, T. Anderson, 'Reasons for Companion Animal Guardianship (Pet Ownership) from Two Populations', *Society and*

Animals, volume 16, issue 3, pp. 279–291, November 2008.

24. A. R. McConnell, et al., 'Friends with benefits: On the positive consequences of pet ownership', *Journal of Personality and Social Psychology*, volume 101, issue 6, pp. 1239–1252, December 2011, DOI: 10.1037/a0024506.

25. BBC News, 'Sudan man forced to "marry" goat', 24 February 2006, news.bbc.co.uk/1/hi/4748292.stm

Chapter 10

1. V. Paquette, et al., '"Change the mind and you change the brain": effects of cognitive-behavioral therapy on the neural correlates of spider phobia', *NeuroImage*, volume 18, issue 2, pp. 401–409, February 2003, ISSN 1053-8119, dx.doi.org/10.1016/S1053-8119(02)00030-7.

2. M. H. Antoni, et al., 'Cognitive-behavioral stress management reverses anxiety-related leukocyte transcriptional dynamics', *Biological Psychiatry*, volume 17, issue 4, pp. 366–372, 15 February 2012, DOI: 10.1016/j.biopsych.2011.10.007.

3. A. T. Spyrou, et al., 'Psychological support and coronary heart disease patients outcomes', *European Heart Journal Supplements*, volume 1, supplement 2, p. 124, 2013.

4. C. B. Becker, E. Stice, *Succeed Body Image Programme Manual*, Oxford University Press, 2011.

5. T. Freijy, E. J. Kothe, 'Dissonance-based interventions for health behaviour change: a systematic review', *British Journal of Health Psychology*, volume18, issue 2, pp. 310–337, 2013.

6. D. Veale, R. Willson, A. Clark, 2009, op. cit.

7. T. F. Cash, *Body Image Workbook*, New Harbinger Publications, 2nd Revised Edition, 2008.

Chapter 11

1. S. L. Michael, et al., 'Parental and Peer Factors Associated with Body Image Discrepancy among Fifth-Grade Boys and Girls', *Journal of Youth and Adolescence*, January 2013, DOI: 10.1007/s 10964-012-9899-8.

References

2. S. Helfert, P. Warshburger, 'A prospective study on the impact of peer and parental pressure on body dissatisfaction in adolescent girls and boys', *Body Image*, volume 8, pp. 101–109, March 2011, dx.doi.org/10.1016/j.bodyim.2011.01.004.

3. R. F. Rodgers, 'Do maternal body dissatisfaction and dietary restraint predict weight gain in young pre-school children? A 1-year follow-up study', *Appetite*, volume 67, pp. 30-36, 2013.

4. L. Sabra, S. L. Katz-Wise, et al., 'Individuation or Identification? Self-Objectification and the Mother–Adolescent Relationship', *Psychology of Women Quarterly*, volume 37, pp. 366–380, September 2013, first published on 14 December 2012, DOI: 10.1177/0361684312468425.

5. A. Taylor, et al., 'Self-esteem and body dissatisfaction in young children: Associations with weight and perceived parenting style', *Clinical Psychologist*, volume 16, pp. 25–35, 2012, DOI: 10.1111/j.1742-9552.2011.00038.x.

6. J. M. Twenge, J. D. Foster, 'Birth Cohort Increases in Narcissistic Personality Traits Among American College Students, 1982–2009', *Social Psychological and Personality Science*, volume 1, issue 1, pp. 99–106.

7. S. H. Konrath, et al., 'Changes in Dispositional Empathy in American College Students Over Time: A Meta-Analysis', *Personality and Social Psychology Review*, volume 15, p. 180, 2011, DOI: 10.1177/1088868310377395.

8. E. Kahana, et al., 2013, op, cit.

9. M. Meeker, *Strong Fathers, Strong Daughters*, Ballantine Books, 2007.

10. L. Chaddock, et al., 'A neuroimaging investigation of the association between aerobic fitness, hippocampal volume, and memory performance in preadolescent children', *Brain Research*, volume 1358, pp. 172–183, 2010.

11. M. A. I. Åberg, et al., 'Cardiovascular fitness is associated with cognition in young adulthood', *PNAS*, volume 106, p. 20906–20911, 2009.

12. G. S. Goldfield, et al., 2012, op. cit.

13. P. Morin, et al., 'Relationship between eating behaviors and physical activity among primary and secondary school students: results of a cross-sectional study', *Journal of School Health*, volume 83, issue 9, pages 597–604, September 2013.

14. Media Smart, 'Body Image Parent Pack', 2012, www.mediasmart.org.uk/parents.

15. A. R. Smith, et al., op. cit.
16. V. Menon, M. Demaray, 2013, op. cit.
17. D. Neumark-Sztainer, 'Family meals and disordered eating in adolescents: longitudinal findings from project EAT', *Archives of Pediatrics & Adolescent Medicine*, volume 162, issue 1, pp. 17–22, 2008.
18. A. J. Hammons, B. H. Fiese, 'Is Frequency of Shared Family Meals Related to the Nutritional Health of Children and Adolescents?', *Pediatrics*, volume 127, issue 6, 2011, DOI: 10.1542/peds.2010-1440.

Chapter 12

1. B. Groves, 'William Banting: The Father of the Low-Carbohydrate Diet', 2002, www.second-opinions.co.uk/banting. html#.Ur_YAmRdXw4.
2. British Dietetic Association, 'Food Fact Sheet: Weight Loss', 2013.
3. L. P. Kozak, 2011, op. cit; P. Seale, 2013, op. cit.
4. C. B. Ebbeling, et al., 'Effects of Dietary Composition on Energy Expenditure During Weight-Loss Maintenance', *JAMA*, volume 307, number 24, pp. 2627–2634, 27 June 2012.
5. D. Ludwig, 'All Calories Not Created Equal, Study Suggests', WebMD Health News, 26 June 2012, www.webmd.com/diet/news/20120626/all-calories-not-created-equal-study-suggests.
6. British Dietetic Association, 'Losing count leads to gaining weight', news statement, Press Centre, 2010.
7. D. E. Larson-Meyer, et al., 'Influence of running and walking on hormonal regulators of appetite in women', *Journal of Obesity*, volume 2012, article ID: 730409, 2012, DOI: 10.1155/2012/730409.
8. C. Martins, et al., 'Effect of chronic exercise on appetite control in overweight and obese individuals', *Medicine & Science in Sports and Exercise*, volume 45, issue 5, pp. 805–812, May 2013, DOI: 10.1249/MSS.0b013e31827d1618.
9. S. A. Plowman, D. L. Smith, *Exercise Physiology for Health Fitness and Performance*, p. 210, 4th Ed, Lippincott Williams & Wilkins, 2013.
10. L. I. Cheikh Ismail, et al., 'Energy and nutrient intakes during dif-

ferent phases of the menstrual cycle in females in the United Arab Emirates', *Annals of Nutrition and Metabolism*, volume 54, issue 2, pp. 124–128, 2009, DOI: 10.1159/000209395.

11. M. Bryant, et al., 'Modest changes in dietary intake across the menstrual cycle: implications for food intake research', *British Journal of Nutrition*, volume 96, issue 5, pp. 888–894, November 2006.

12. Bupa, '1 in 5 Brits admit to not leaving their desk all day', News Centre Release, 17 October 2013.

13. R. J. van de Laar, et al., 'Self-reported time spent watching television is associated with arterial stiffness in young adults: the Amsterdam Growth and Health Longitudinal Study', British Journal of Sports Medicine, published first online on 7 October 2013, DOI: 10.1136/bjsports-2013-092555 2013.

14. A. Sigman, 'Time for a view on screen time', *Archives of Disease in Childhood*, volume 9, issue 11, pp. 935–942, DOI: 10.1136/archdischild-2012-302196.

15. D. M. Jackson, et al., 'Increased television viewing is associated with elevated body fatness but not with lower total energy expenditure in children', *American Journal of Clinical Nutrition*, volume 89, issue 4, pp. 1031–1036, 2009.

16. C. Fitzpatrick, et al., 'Early Childhood Television Viewing Predicts Explosive Leg Strength And Waist Circumference By Middle Childhood', *International Journal of Behavioral Nutrition and Physical Activity*, volume 9, issue 87, 16 July 2012, DOI: 10.1186/1479-5868-9-87.

17. TV Licensing, 'The changing ways we're watching the box', 2011, www.tvlicensing.co.uk/resources/library/BBC/MEDIA_CENTRE/TeleScope_infographic.pdf.

18. C. D. Summerbell, H. J. Moore, ToyBox-study group, et al., 'Evidence-based recommendations for the development of obesity prevention programs targeted at preschool children', *Obesity Reviews*, volume 13, pp. 129–132, 2012, DOI: 10.1111/ j.1467-789X.2011.00940.x.

19. D. J. Hruschka, et al., 'Shared Norms and Their Explanation for the Social Clustering of Obesity', *American Journal of Public Health*, volume 101, supplement 1, 2011.

20. N. A. Christakis. J. H. Fowler, 'The Spread of Obesity in a Large Social Network over 32 Years', *New England Journal of Medicine*, volume 357, pp. 370–379, 2007.

21. D. J. Hruschka, et al., 2011, op. cit.

22. Academy Of Medical Royal Colleges, 'Measuring Up: The Medical Profession's Prescription For The Nation's Obesity Crisis', February 2013.
23. E. V. Carraca, et al. 'Body image change and improved eating self-regulation in a weight management intervention in women', *International Journal of Behavioral Nutrition and Physical Activity*, volume 8, issue 75, 2011, www.ijbnpa.org/content/8/1/75.

Chapter 13

1. D. K. Keith, 'Body Image Education as a Prevention Measure for eating Disorders in Ninth-Grade Students', All Graduate Theses and Dissertations, paper 758, 2010, digitalcommons.usu.edu/etd/758.
2. HM Government, 'Response to the consultation – Building a fairer Britain: reform of the Equality and Human Rights Commission', Government Equalities Office, 15 May 2012, Crown Copyright.
3. Creative Diversity Network, 'The CDN Mandate', 2013.
4. Royal College of Psychiatrists, 'Eating Disorders Section: Statement on the influence of the media on eating disorders', February 2010.
5. BMA Board of Science and Education statement, 'BMA demands more responsible media attitude on body image', *British Medical Journal*, volume 320, issue 7248, p. 1495, 2000.
6. M. A. Lelwica, *The Religion of Thinness*, Gürze Books LLC, 2009.
7. Ibid.

Appendix A

1. N. Trefethen, Revised BMI calculator, 2013, people.maths.ox.ac.uk/trefethen/bmi_calc.html.
2. A. Oreopoulos, et al., 'More on Body Fat Cutoff Points–Reply–I', *Mayo Clinic Proceedings*, volume 86, issue 6, pp. 584–585, June 2011, DOI: 10.4065/mcp.2011.0156.

Resources

There are times when body dissatisfaction may be one aspect of a deeper, more complex problem such as anorexia, bulimia, binge-eating disorder or body dysmorphic disorder.

Screening

Screening 'quizzes' are not diagnostic tests, nor can they provide you with a diagnosis but they may help to identify symptoms of concern that are having a significant impact on your life. A valid and reliable diagnosis can only be made in partnership with your doctor or mental health professional.

The Body Dysmorphic Disorder Program at Rhode Island Hospital has a confidential online self-screening test for either adults or adolescents: www.rhodeislandhospital.org/services/body-dysmorphic-disorder-program/questionnaires.html.

The Eating Attitudes Test is an example of a self-administered screening questionnaire for eating issues: psychcentral.com/quizzes/eat.htm.

Professional help

If you feel you need professional help with eating or body image issues, in the UK your doctor is usually the first and best port of call. Doctors are normally aware of local services.

If you want help more quickly and want to seek private help the national organisations below may be able to recommend someone suitable. You can also try to find an accredited therapist. For example, you can contact The British Association for Behavioural and Cognitive Psychotherapies (BABCP) via the 'Find a CBT Therapist' section on their website, www.babcp.com.

Eating Disorders

UK

NHS CHOICES
Website:
www.nhs.uk/Conditions/Anorexia-nervosa/Pages/Symptoms.aspx

BEAT provides helplines, online support and a network of UK-wide self-help groups to help adults and young people in the UK overcome their eating disorders.
Website: www.b-eat.co.uk/get-help/
Helpline: 0845 634 1414

Australia

The Eating Disorders Association Inc
Website: eda.org.au/
Tel: (07) 3394 3661

New Zealand

Eating Disorders Association of New Zealand (EDANZ)
Website: www.ed.org.nz
Free Phone: 0800 2 EDANZ

Body Dysmorphic Disorder (BDD)

UK

NHS CHOICE BDD
Website:
www.nhs.uk/Conditions/body-dysmorphia/ Pages/Introduction.
aspx

The BDD Foundation
Website: www.thebddfoundation.com/what_isbdd/whatisbdd1.
htm

BDD Help
Website: www.bddhelp.co.uk

Further Reading

D. Veale, R. Willson, A. Clark, *Overcoming Body Image Problems Including Body Dysmorphic Disorder*, Constable & Robinson: London, 2009.

T. F. Cash, *Body Image Workbook*, New Harbinger Publications, 2008.

S. Wilhelm, *Feeling Good About the Way You Look*, Guilford Press; New Edition, 2006.

Basics Of Nutrition And Weight Loss

British Dietetic Association (BDA) Food Facts sheets about many aspects of nutrition are free to download and print from www.bda.uk.com/foodfacts.

The BDA also has a dedicated website for weight loss: www.bdaweight-wise.com.

NHS Choices: www.nhs.uk/livewell/loseweight/Pages/Loseweighthome.aspx.

The US National Institute of Health, Weight-control Information Network has a wide variety of free booklets and fact sheets to view or download at win.niddk.nih.gov/publications/index.htm.

Further Reading
Becoming More Physically Active

Excellent free information on how to become more physically active is available in the Mental Health Foundation's 'Let's Get Physical: The impact of physical activity on well being', 2013: www.mentalhealth.org.uk/content/assets/PDF/publications/lets-get-physical-report.pdf?view=Standard.

NHS Choices, Get Active Your way: www.nhs.uk/Livewell/fitness/Pages/Activelifestyle.aspx.

'Tips to get you Active', US Department Of Health And Human Services, National Institutes of Health. NIH Publication No. 06–5578, September 2013: win.niddk.nih.gov/publications/tips.htm.

Index

Note: page numbers in **bold** refer to illustrations.

achievement 6–8, 79–80
actresses, permarexic 50
Adatto, Rachel 50
ADHD *see* attention deficit hyperactivity
    disorder
advertising 17, 179
ageism 174–5, 205–6
aggression, teenage 134
Aguilera, Christina 96
airbrushing 16, 50, 61
Aird, Rosemary 127
Alba, Jessica 95
alcohol consumption 5, 31, 162, 189, 192
altruism 152
American Journal of Public Health 128,
    153, 196
American Psychological Association 13,
    80
amygdala 58
anabolic steroids 4, 111–13
ancient art 87–8
android body-fat distribution 29, **29**, 33,
    35
    see also apple-shaped women
Aniston, Jennifer 54, 62
anorexia nervosa ix, 12, 15
    and athletes 38
    death rate 13
    and peer body weight 10
    psychological therapies for 165
    social transmission 168
anterior cingulate cortex 154–5
anthropometry 36

anxiety 57–8, 63, 133, 136, 140, 154–5,
    161
Appearance & Performance Enhancing
    Drugs (APEDs) 112–13
    see also anabolic steroids
appetite 26–7, 190–1
Appetite (journal) 20–1, 168
apple-shaped women 29, 43, 212
    see also android body-fat distribution
Archives of Disease in Childhood 193–4
Archives of Sexual Behavior 72
arterial stiffening 193
Asian Journal of Andrology 108
Asian people 112
Asian-American people 49
assimilation 54
atheism 155
atherosclerosis 135
athletes 37–9, 112, 129
attachment theory 89–90
attention
    body bias 125–6
    economy 126–33
    fatigue 131
    'outwards' focused 125–7, 152, 154,
        156, 158, 170–1, 199, 200
    parental 169
    restoration through nature 130–2
    self-focused 125–7, 152, 154, 156,
        158, 170–1, 199
attention deficit hyperactivity disorder
    (ADHD) 128–9
attractiveness 60–1

Index

autistic traits 14

baby blues 89–90
Banting, William 184
BAT *see* brown adipose tissue
BBC *see* British Broadcasting
 Corporation
BBW *see* Big Beautiful Woman
beauty advertisements 38
belly barging 114–15
belonging, sense of 154, 155
Bhutan 47
Bidayuh people 149–50
Big Beautiful Woman (BBW) 83
'bigorexia' 104–5
binge-eating 31
binge-eating disorder 12, 165
bioelectrical impedance analysis (BIA) 36
biofeedback-assisted autogenic training
 133
Biological Psychiatry (journal) 57
bisexual women, sexual preferences 71–2,
 85
BJU International (journal) 107–8
blindness 44–5, 68
blood pressure levels 158
  see also hypertension
blood-fat levels 28, 188
blood-sugar (glucose) levels 5, 28, 187–8
body building 4, 102–3, 111–12
body comparisons 19–20, 52–3
body competition 10, 18–19
Body Confidence Campaign 203
body dissatisfaction ix–xiv, 3–9
  and the attention economy 126–33
  and attentional body bias 125–6
  and careers 18–19
  causes of 9–21
  commonplace nature 4
  effects of 5–9
  and exposure to thin body ideals 44–63
  and locus of control 133–4
  and male desire 64–86
  and manorexia 55, 102–15
  and materialism 19–21
  as normative discontent 3, 198–9
  and optimal desired body size 22–43
  as pain 124–5
  parental transmission of 166–82
  and pregnancy 87–101
  requiring psychological intervention 120
  and the Slenderati 16–18
  and status aspiration 18–19
  see also combating body dissatisfaction

body fascism 85
body hair removal 114
body image ix, xi–xii
  of children 169, 171, 175–9
  and dieting 40–1
  of immigrants 49
  male disorders 55
  and mother–daughter relationships 32
  and online social comparison–making
   147
  and physical exercise 137, 138–9
  and psychological therapies 163–4
  and socially transmitted cultural ideals
   119
  and weight loss 197
body language 80, 81, 82
Body Mass Index (BMI) 9, 34–5, 36, 49–
 50, 72, 183, 194
  calculation 209–12
  and frame size 209
  interpretation 211–12
  of our friends 196
  and percentage body-fat 213
  Z score 168
body satisfaction
  promotion 121
  see also body dissatisfaction
body shape
  as measure of health 34, 35
  see also apple-shaped women; pear-
   shaped women
body size, optimal desired 22–43
  and appetite traits 26–7
  and the diet industry 40–1
  and extreme physical fitness 37–9
  and foetal programming 25–6
  and genetics 24–30, 42
  and hormones 28, 32–3
  maternal influences on 32
  and NEAT 27
  and 'obesogenic' environments 25, 41–3
  and personality 31–2
  reality checks regarding 33–6
body weight xi
  control 14
  genetically programmed baseline 27
  and guilt 21
  as measure of health 33–6
  perceived 5, 10, 23
  see also body size, optimal desired;
    body-fat; obesity; overweight;
    underweight; weight loss; weight
    regain
body dysmorphic disorder 165

body-fat
  brown 30, 185, 186
  effects of losing 185, 186
  and the endocrine system 185
  facts 186–97
  primary function of 74
  white 30, 185, 186
body-fat distribution 27–30, 33
  android/apple-shaped women 29, **29**,
    33, 35, 43, 212
  discussing with children 172
  and ethnicity 30
  and genetics 24–5, 27–30
  gynoid (pear-shaped women) xii, 9–10,
    24, 28, **29**, 35, 212
  and over-exercising 14–16
  uneven nature 192
body-fat percentage 35–6, 183, 213
Body-image Resilience Model 120–1
body-shaping behaviours 52–3
bone density 34–5, 37, 38
boredom 126
bottom(s)
  fat xii, 66–7, 69, 172
  see also buttocks
boys
  body building 4
  puberty 172–3
  see also manorexia
brain 81, 124, 136
  children's 177–8
  and cognitive behavioural therapy 161
  and fame 61–2
  gender differences in 55–9, 70–1
  and religion 154–5
  rewiring the 161
Brain Research (journal) 177
Braithwaite, Binky 115
Brazil, Bobo 102
breast 66
  cancer 6, 161
  development 172
  implants 85
  shape 92
  size 72–3, 74–5, 85
breastfeeding 89, 91–2, 95
British Broadcasting Corporation (BBC)
  204–5
*British Journal of Developmental
  Psychology* 3
British Journal of Urology International
  107
brown adipose tissue (BAT) 30, 185, 186
Bruni, Carla 94

Bryson, Bill 77
Buddhists 514
bulimia nervosa 12, 15, 38, 165
bulimic symptoms 147
'bumpophilia' 94
Bupa Ground Miles campaign 193
buttock(s)
  fat 28, 35, 70
  size 72–3
  see also bottoms

C-reactive protein 153
calories, unequal nature 187–9
cancer 6, 35, 135, 161, 212
carbohydrates 187
cardiovascular disease 28, 40, 135, 153
cardiovascular fitness 177
careers 18–19
caring people 77–80, 151–3, 171, 192, 200
Catherine, Duchess of Cambridge 93–4,
  96
Catholics 154
CBT see cognitive-behavioural therapy
CDN see Creative Diversity Network
celebrities
  overweight 62–3
  slender 54, 57, 61–3, 201–2
    celebrity mums 93–6
    diets 15–16
    exercise regimes 142–3
    fascination with 61
    over-exercising compulsions 15–16
    personally relevant 61–2
Cell Metabolism (journal) 25
cellulite 93
character 31–2
charitable donations 152
chick-lit 11–12
children
  and ageism 174–5
  and body dissatisfaction 166–82
  discussing puberty with 171–3
  healthy eating habits 178–9
  and mastery experiences 170
  and 'media literacy' 17, 179–81, 201
  obese 177, 178, 195
  objectification of 182
  and 'outwards' focused attention 170–1
  overweight 178
  and physical activity 177–9
  role modelling for 173–4, 176
  and screen time 194, 195, 200
  and social comparison-making 173
China 14

Index

Chinese tradition 83
chocolate 20–1
choice 42, 143–4
cholesterol levels 158
Christianity 153
'Chubby Chasers' 82–3
Clements, Kirstie 85–6
coach potatoes 193–5
cognitive eating 12, 200
cognitive-behavioural therapy (CBT) 160–1, 163–5
combating body dissatisfaction 119–207
  in children 166–82
  and dieting 183–97
  paradigm shift 123–34
  and physical exercise 135–44
  and psychological therapies 160–5
  and social relationships 145–59
Combs, Sean 'P. Diddy' x
common experiences 156–7
competency, sense of 134, 144
computer games 105–6, 151
consumption 200
contrast effect 61
control 170
  locus of 133–4, 158
  need for 14
  perception of 124
  self-control 155
cortisol 188
cosmetics industry 114
cravings 192
Creative Diversity Network (CDN) 203–4
Crimmins, Cathy 98
Cyrus, Miley 54
Czech Republic 13

Daily Mash (satirical website) 84
Dayak people 108
death, risk of
  and anorexia nervosa 13
  and psychological therapies 161
  and social relationships 146–7
depression 126, 133, 135–6
  antenatal 90, 139–40
  'Facebook Depression' 60, 150
  postnatal 89–90
deprivation, relative 20
diabetes 28, 134, 135
  type-2 29, 35, 212
Dick the Bruiser 102
diet industry 40–1, 183
dieting 183–97
  failure 53, 183, 184–5

low-carb diets 184, 188
low-fat diets 188
low-GI diets 188–9
Messiah diets 184
physical consequences of 185
and the thin media ideal 52–3
yo-yo 40
disability, chronic 154
dissonance-based interventions 160–1, 162–3
distraction 124–5, 131
diversional therapy 134
diversity issues 203–5
dog ownership 158, 159
DPC Scale 8
dress size xi

Eastern Europe, Westernization 13
eating disorder not otherwise specified (EDNOS) 12, 38
eating disorders 12–14, 202, 206
  and athletes 37–8
  causes 14, 17–18
  dissonance-based interventions for 162
  in Fiji 46
  and the gendered brain 58, 59
  in Israeli society 50
  and over-exercising 15
  and postnatal depression 89
  psychological therapies for 162, 165
  role of the media in 17–18, 51
  and social comparison-making 57
  see also specific eating disorders
eating habits
  eating cognitively 12, 200
  healthy 178–9, 184, 185
Ebbeling, Carl 188
'eight-packs' 113
emotional baggage 123
empathy 70, 171
endocannabinoids 136
endocrine system 185
endorphins 178
epigenetics 25–6
equality issues 203–5
ethnicity 30
Evolution and Human Behaviour (journal) 68
eye-to-eye contact 149

face-to-face interaction 148–51
Facebook 171
  'Facebook Depression' 60, 150
  maladaptive usage 147–9

fame 62
family connectedness 145–6, 182
family mealtimes 182
fashion editors 16–18, 85–6
fashion models 49–50, 54
'fat talk' 11
father–daughter relationships 175–7
fathers 88–9
fear 57, 58
Female Athlete Triad 38
feminism 71–2
fertility indicators 70, 71
fertility symbols 87–8
Fiji 46
Fink, Dr Bernhard 81
fitness instructors 142–3
foetus
    development 70, 71
    programming 25–6
food
    fetish 12
    intake control 14
    your relationship with 12
foreign cultures 45–50
frame size, calculation 208–9
free will 42
friends, body weight of 9–10, 195–6
frontal lobes 178
functional magnetic resonance imaging
    (fMRI) 81, 124

gait, attractiveness of 81
gay men 66
gaze, male xii
Geary, D. C. 80
genetics 201
    and appetite traits 26–7
    and body-fat distribution 24–5, 27–30
    and muscle mass 104
    and overweight 24–30, 32, 42
    social influences on 147
gerontophobia 174–5
gestalt effect 76
ghrelin 26, 190
GI see glycaemic index
Giffin, Emily 11–12
Glaser, Sherry 98
gluteofemoral fat (fat of the hips, thighs
    and buttocks) xii, 28, 30, 35, 66–70,
    172, 192
glycaemic index (GI) 187–9
God 154–5
Gordimer, Nadine 64
government support 202–3

greenery, exposure to 128–33
guilt 21
Guthman, Julie 42
gynoid body-fat distribution (pear-shaped
    women) xii, 9–10, 24, 28, 29, 35, 212

Hadza hunter–gatherers 73
handbags 20
Harvard Business Review 126
heart attack 153
heart disease 35, 158, 161, 188, 212
high-fat diets 25
Hilfiger, Tommy x
hippocampus 62, 177
hips
    fat xii, 28, 30, 35, 66–70, 172
    phobia 85
Holmes, Katie 95
hormones 112
    and appetite control 190
    female 28, 32–3, 70
human growth hormone 112
hypertension 35, 212

ideals
    muscular/'ripped' 103, 104–6, 111–13,
        167, 172–3
    thin body 44–63, 92, 119, 132, 160–1,
        162, 207
    see also celebrities, slender
ill health, chronic 154
immigrants 49
immune system 135, 161
impulsivity 31
in vitro fertilisation (IVF) 100
Independent (newspaper) 115
individualism, cult of 127, 171
institutional support 202–3
insulin resistance 29, 134, 188
intellectual capacity 135–6, 177
Intellectual Quotient (IQ) 177
interleukin 6 153
International Body Project 4
International Journal of Eating Disorders
    3–4
International Journal of Happiness and
    Development 152
Internet
    displacement effects 149–51
    social media 147–51, 171, 179–80
intimacy satisfaction 89
Inzlicht, Michael 155
Israel 49–50
IVF see in vitro fertilisation

Index

Japan 14
Jewish people 154
Journal of Affective Disorders 147
Journal of the American Medical Association 187–8
Journals of Gerontology 134
Jung, Carl 145

Karan, Donna x
Kardashian, Kim 96
Klum, Heidi 95
Korea 108

Lancet (journal) 42, 131
Large Passions 82
Lauren, Ralph x
leg(s)
    fat 70
    see also thigh(s)
lesbian women, sexual preferences 10, 71–2, 85
life issues, avoidance of 123–4
'locker-room' syndrome 109
locus of control 133–4, 158
loneliness 158
Lopez, Jennifer 95
love, unconditional 181
Ludwig, David 188

'male gaze' xii
manorexia 55, 102–15
    and belly barging 114–15
    and the cosmetics industry 114
    'eight-packs' 113
    and the muscular/'ripped' ideal 103, 104–6, 111–13, 167, 172–3
    and negative appearance-related comments 114
    and penis size 106–10
    'six-packs' 111–13
mastery experiences 133, 138, 170, 178
materialism 19–21
MDM *see* muscle dysmorphia
mealtimes
    family 182
    in front of the TV 195
media
    advertising 17, 179
    chick-lit 11–12
    high levels of exposure to 59–60
    idealised slender body image of 44–63, 132
    lack of reality-based imagery 204–7
    and manorexia 105–6, 108, 109–10
    and 'media literacy' 17, 179–81, 201, 203
    and pregnancy/early motherhood 93–4
media-mom columnists 98–9
medial prefrontal cortex (mPFC) 58–9
men 55–9
    'Chubby Chasers' 82–3
    with low waist-to-hip ratios 69
    and the 'male gaze' xii
    and the 'redundant male' concept 56
    role in combating body dissatisfaction 175–7, 202
    sexual preferences of 64–86
    see also manorexia
Mendick, Heather 37
menopause 28, 33
Men's Health magazine 113
menstrual cycle 76, 192
menstruation, absent/infrequent 38
mental health 136–8
metabolic rate 33, 185
micropenis 108
Mind (charity) 6
mindfulness 614
models 49–50, 54
moisturisers, male 114
mood boosters 135, 136
mother–adolescent relationship 169
mother–baby attachment 89–90
mother–daughter relationship 32
mothers 87–101
    body image of 168
    celebrity mums 93–4
    effects of the maternal diet in pregnancy 25–6
    full-time 96–7
    and maternal role-modelling 101
    media-mom columnists 98–9
    obese 64
    and the politicisation of motherhood 97–8
    rebirth 99–101
mPFC *see* medial prefrontal cortex
Müller, Manfred J. 28
muscle dysmorphia (MDM) 104–5
muscle mass 34–5
    'eight-packs' 113
    and genetics 104
    loss of 33
    muscle-enhancing strategies 102, 105, 111–12
    muscular/'ripped' ideals 103, 104–6, 111–13, 167, 172–3
    and resistance training 191

muscle mass – *continued*
  'six-packs' 4, 37, 111–13
  'virtual' muscularity 105–6
music 124–5
Muslims 154

narcissism 170–1
nature 128–33
NeuroImage (journal) 56–7
neuroticism 31, 154
New England Journal of Medicine 196
New Spirituality 127
newsreaders, permarexic 50–1
Ngedup, Sangay 48
non-exercise activity thermogenesis
  (NEAT) 27
non-verbal communication 80, 81–2
norepinephrine 136, 178
normative discontent 3, 198–9
norms, slender xiii
novelty-seeking 31
nurses 77
nurturing 77–80

obesity
  and BMI 211
  causes of 186
  central 29
  childhood 177, 178, 195
  epidemic 42
  and foetal programming 26
  friends with 195–6
  and genetics 25, 26, 28, 29, 30, 32
  and pear-shaped women 28
  and personality 31–2
  and pet ownership 158
  and pregnancy 90–1
  prevalence 64
  and technology 193
Obesity Research (journal) 30
'obesogenic' environment 25, 41–3, 195,
  197, 201
objectification
  of children 182
  see also self-objectification
Observer magazine 4
Observer newspaper 39
oestrogen 28, 33, 70
old age 3–4, 174–5
O'Leary, Michael 107
Olympic Games, 2012 37–9
opiates/opioids 136
orgasm 8–9
osteoporosis 35, 38

Otis, Carré 15–16
'outwards' focused attention 125–7, 152,
  154, 156, 158, 170–1, 199, 200
overweight
  and BMI 211
  causes of 186
  and children 178
  friends/peers 9–10
  and pregnancy 90–1
  prevalence 64
  see also obesity
ovulation, non-verbal signs of 81–2

pain 124–5
parents
  attention 169
  influence on body dissatisfaction 166–
    82
  as role models 167, 173–4, 176, 180,
    202
  support 181–2
pear-shaped women (gynoid) xii, 9–10,
  24, 28, **29**, 35, 212
  male preferences for 68–70
Pediatrics (journal) 153
peers, body weight of 9–10, 195–6
penile augmentation surgery 108, 110
penile dysmorphic disorder 107–8
penis response profiling 65–6
penis size 106–10
pensioners 3–4
percentage body-fat 35–6, 183, 213
perception 17, 57–8
  of body weight 5, 10, 23
  of control 124
perfectionism 14
perimenopause 32–3
permarexia 50–1, 207
personal attractiveness 60–1
personality type 31–2
pets 157–9
phone sex 76–7
physical exercise 135–44, 200
  choice of 143–4
  chronic 190–1
  and the dangers of the extreme 'toned
    and fit' appearance 52
  and fitness instructors 142–3
  lack of 6, 193, 193–5
  making time for 143–4
  and nature 129–30
  over-exercising 14–16
  physical effects of 135
  and pregnancy 139–40

Index

psychological effects of 135–40, 144
recommended levels of 140–1
resistance training 191
Roman views on 141–2
and sexual functioning 9
social anxieties regarding 141
spot reduction 191–2
and weight control 186, 189–92
physical fitness 37–9
Plowman, Sharon 192
pornography 108, 109–10
postnatal
  body 88–9, 93–6, 100
  depression 89–90
prefrontal cortex 58–9
pregnancy xiii, 64, 87–8, 90–4, 99–100
  antenatal depression 90, 139–40
  celebrity mums 93–4
  and maternal diet 25–6
  and overweight/obese 90–1
  and physical exercise 139–40
  teenage 174
pro-social spending 152
Proceedings of the National Academy of Sciences 177
professional achievement 7–8
Protestants 154
Psychological Science (journal) 81–2, 155
psychological therapies 160–5
  cognitive-behavioural techniques 160–1, 163–5
  dissonance-based interventions 160–1, 162–3
Psychology of Men & Masculinity (journal) 113–14
Psychology of Women Quarterly (journal) 72
puberty 171–3
public education programmes 201

Quetelet, Adolphe 209

Red Cross 134
relationships 8
  father–daughter 175–7
  feminine skills 80–1
  with food 12
  friendships 9–10, 195–6
  mother–adolescent 169
  mother–baby 89–90
  mother–daughter 32
  and physical exercise 137
  romantic 18–19

social support 145–59
relative deprivation 20
relaxation training 164
religion 153–6, 207
resource availability 74–5
role models
  for children 173–4, 176
  female 16, 17, 37, 39, 142, 180
  parental 167, 173–4, 176, 180, 202
romantic relationships 18–19
Roosevelt, Theodore 44
Ryan, Richard 132

Sadhu people 108
Sarkozy, Nicolas 94
satiety 194–5
schizophrenia 136
Schwarzenegger, Arnold 28, 102
screen time 150–1, 193–5, 200
secondary sexual characteristics 66, 76, 172
secular society 153, 207
sedentary lifestyles 6, 193, 193–5
self, cult of the 127, 171, 200
self-control 155
self-esteem
  children's 168, 175
  gender differences in 56
  and Internet use 151
  and penis size 106
  and pet ownership 158
  and physical exercise 137, 138, 143
self-focused attention 125–7, 152, 154, 156, 158, 170–1, 199
self-objectification 7–8
self-worth 152, 168
Seneca 141–2
sex lines 76–7
sexual dimorphism 69–71
sexual health 5–6, 162
sexual satisfaction 8–9
Shangri-la 47–8
shoes 20
Sigman, Professor 72–3
'six-packs' 4, 37, 111–13
'size-zero' culture 39
sizeism 205–6
Slenderati 16–18
'small-penis syndrome' 108
smell, sense of 81–2
Smith, April R. 18–19
Smith, Denise L. 192
smoking 5, 16, 162
soaps, slimming 55

257

social comparison-making 19, 56–7, 60–3
  male 56
  on-line 147, 179–80
  self-critical 56
  see also body comparisons
social isolation 147
social media 171
  as antisocial networking 147–51, 179–80
  displacement effects 149–51
social norms
  normative discontent 3, 198–9
  slender xiii
  social-norm hypothesis 195–6
social support 145–59
  and caring for others 151–3
  and common experiences 156–7
  parental 181–2
  and pets 157–9
  and religion 153–6
  and social networking 147–51
Society and Animals (journal) 158
socioeconomic background 74–5
Spain 50–1
spending, pro-social 152
spirituality 127, 153–6
spot reduction 191–2
startle responses 59
status 61
  aspiration 18–19
steroids, anabolic 4, 111–13
stress 161
stretch marks 93
stroke 28, 153, 188
structure, sense of 159
subconscious mind 179, 201
subcutaneous fat 28
suicide 13
Super-size Big Beautiful Woman (SSBBW) 83

Taylor, Shelley 80–1
teasing 114, 176–7
teenage violence/aggression 134
television 60, 193–5, 203–4
television presenters, permarexic 50
temperament 31–2
testosterone 82, 103, 104, 173
thermogenic fat strippers 113
thigh(s)
  fat xii, 28, 30, 35, 66–7, 69–70, 172
  phobia 85

thin body ideal 44–63, 119, 132, 207
  and pregnancy 92
  psychological therapies to combat 160–1, 162
  see also celebrities, slender
thin women, and body dissatisfaction 4
'thinspiration' 44–63
Time magazine 95
tissue-eating 86
Tombe, Charles 159
'toned and fit' appearance, extreme 52
Tonga 41, 45
Topinama people 108
tummies
  fat 192
  workouts 191–2
  see also waist fat

unconditional love 181
underweight
  and BMI 211
  and body dissatisfaction 3
  fashion models 49–50
urbanisation 130–1

values 174
Venus of Laussel 88
Venus of Willendorf 87–8
videophilia 132
violence, teenage 134
'virtual' muscularity 105–6
visual impairment 44–5
Vogue Australia 85–6
voices, female 76–7
volunteering 152, 153

waist fat 28, 30, 33, 35
waist-to-buttocks (WTB) ratio 72
waist-to-hip (WTH) ratio 35, 68, 69–70, 72, 183
  calculation 212
Walker, Laura Jensen 11–12
Washington, George xi
weight cycling 40
weight loss
  postnatal 95–6
  smoking for 5, 16
  successful 183–4
weight regain 40, 185
white adipose tissue (WAT) 30, 185, 186
World Health Organization (WHO) 4, 91, 186